I GOT THIS

Becoming a Warrior for Your Own Health

SHELAH DAVIS

I looked up at her beautiful hazel eyes; mine filled with tears. "I am so sorry."

"For what?" she whispered.

"For not being able to fix you, Momma."

She reached up and stroked my face with her hand. She told me that she loved me and tried again to convince me that it wasn't my battle.

That was one of the last cognitive moments that I had with my Mom before cancer consumed her body and took her from all of us.

At the time, what she didn't realize is that I had already waged war: against her cancer. Against my uncle's cancer. Against the diabetes that took my various Aunts and Uncles. Against the cancer that took my grandpa. The heart disease that had almost taken my Dad. The migraines that plagued my friends. The arthritis that crippled my elders.

I had knowledge that would help others who were fighting cancer, diabetes, heart disease, arthritis, high blood pressure and many other diseases. It could save their own daughters from having the moment that I was having in that Hospice center. It could save them from the diseases that would cause them pain and potentially take their lives.

Oh yes. It was war. And the moment that my Momma took her last breath – it was on!

Here is to all of my Health Warriors. May you be armed so that you can fight for your own health and the health of your families..

In 2006, I weighed roughly 253 pounds. I say roughly because at 253, I stopped stepping on the scale. That same year, I lost two close family members to cancer. Somewhere in the midst of the chaos of raising three small babies, working from home, and launching a new marriage, I landed myself in the ER. I thought for certain that I had inherited the heart disease that plagued my father. I also thought the ER trip was due to the fact that I was having a heart attack and would soon become one of those awful statistics. I recall laying on the hospital bed, tears streaming down my face, thinking to myself that if I could just be handed a do-over, I would make it right.

The young doctor walked in and informed me that I was, in fact, not having a heart attack; I was having panic attacks. They handed me a prescription for Zanax and sent me on my merry way. So, I wasn't unhealthy, just a mental case, but more importantly: I had indeed been handed my do over.

That wake up call was just what I needed. I struggled for months trying to not feel like a crazy lady. In doing so, I began noticing that just about everything I read about anxiety/panic disorder could be improved with diet...not drugs. I also noticed that dietary changes were directly tied to recovery from and the curing of many major diseases and conditions. Cancer, heart disease, M.S., chrohns, diabetes, arthritis, high blood pressure...you get the idea.

So my journey began.

In the coming years, I lost more family to cancer but I made DRASTIC changes to my life:

- ✓ I stopped eating meat.
- ✓ I stopped drinking soda.
- ✓ I cut back my caffeine intake.
- ✓ I stopped eating processed sugar.
- ✓ I began exercising seriously.
- ✓ I took serious control of my stress management.

Here is what happened to me as a result of those changes that I made without the help of a physician, a nutritionist or a personal trainer:

I lost over 90 pounds without really even trying.

I no longer had to rely on or take prescription medication for my anxiety disorder.

My fingernails, hair, and skin looked better than they ever had before.

I was full of energy.

I reduced my risk of developing heart disease, cancer, and diabetes by over 75%.

I wasn't plagued with colds or sinus issues any more.

My joints quit aching and I felt more youthful.

I met some incredible people who continue to inspire me every single day.

Thanks to my Momma, I found the balls I needed to write a fricken book to tell anyone who will read it how THEY can take charge of their own lives, their own health, and their own happiness.

There are so many products currently on the market claiming to be THE way to lose weight and be healthy. There are shakes, drinks, exercise programs, magic pills...it's no wonder it is so mind boggling. I am here to tell you that it doesn't have to be so damn complicated to drop the excess pounds or to find optimal health. Honest.

There is one big thing that I will ask of you, dear reader, as you journey on through this book:

FORGET EVERYTHING THAT YOU HAVE BEEN TOLD ABOUT FOOD UP TO THIS POINT.

The reason that I ask this of you? For the past couple of decades, we have had a countless number of miracle cures for our chunky asses and beer bellies crammed right down our throats..."professionals" and celebrities alike all claiming that their way is the way to be healthy and live longer. There are companies who are trying to convince you that you can continue to eat crap as long as you sprinkle it with their magic powder before hand. There are pills that speed up your metabolism so that the pounds just melt away. There are trainers who give you the perfect combination of exercises to do, the perfect numbers of sets so that your body burns the optimum amount of fat cells right off of those "problem areas." I could go on and on, however, I would prefer to get to the solution. The REAL solution.

Listen closely because I am about to tell you how you can reach your optimum health. It doesn't take pills nor are you required to hire a personal trainer. Hell, you don't even have to join a gym. Ready? Here it is, in as plain of a version of English as I can muster for you. The secret to reaching optimal health and being able to call yourself a Health Warrior:

Take in an adequate amount of proper calories each day and don't eat garbage!

Really. That is all there is to it. Sounds easy right? You will have to pardon my sarcasm but really, it IS that simple. Wait, you expected more than that when you picked up this book? Oh alright. Let's get started.

Chapter 1

Is This BS?

The voyage of discovery is not in seeking new landscapes but in having new eyes.
Marcel Proust

During my health journey, I have had the pleasure of studying under some of the greatest minds in the field of fitness and nutrition. T. Collin Campbell, Dr. Neal Barnard, Dr. Caldwell Esselstyn, Rory Freedman, Bill Tara, Dr. Janet Konefal and many others. I have been fortunate enough to sit in on lectures, read their books, attend their seminars, study their findings and I have even joined them while traversing the blue waters of the Caribbean. It humbles me to think about having the opportunity to learn from them and people like them. That alone doesn't qualify me to make decisions that affect YOUR health, however. What qualifies me to make decisions that affect your health is absolutely nothing.

You see, I am of the belief that health is a personal journey. Those decisions aren't any more mine than they should be that of your doctor. It is after all YOUR body. Right?

What we eat affects us all differently. Treatments affect us differently. Some of us have allergies to certain things. Some will have children or jobs that elevate their stress levels. Some won't have access to certain foods to help treat specific conditions and sometimes, just sometimes, you might realize that something you read is just a big old pile of shit.

So, how can you know if what I am putting in front of you isn't among that pile of shit?

You can take the advice of some of the best names in nutrition research and ask yourself a couple of very simple questions:

1. *Does what you are reading/seeing make sense?* You have to be able to shut off any preconceived notions about things you might have been programmed to believe in the past and look at what is in your face right now. Can you understand it or is it a bunch of big words that requires a PHD for you to even begin to comprehend? Because if you are reading it, and you can't make sense of it, how on earth can you even begin to believe it, let alone begin to implement the teachings into your own life? Find a source that speaks the same language that you do. If you have a PHD, then more scientific study will probably appeal to you just fine but if you are a regular person without a huge scientific background, you would probably appreciate gathering your information from reliable sources that are straight forward and easier to swallow. (Hopefully that is also what brought you to be holding THIS particular book.)

2. *Is it true?* Can all of this stuff be proven somehow or does it go on the basis of a lot of smoke and mirrors? Nutrition is science. Science can be proven. Period. If it can't be proven, that means that it is most likely someone's opinion and you know what they say about those don't you? If it can be proven, then take the time to seek the proof either from the one speaking it or from other reliable sources. (My sources are very neatly organized at the end of this book for your perusing enjoyment.)

3. *Does this matter?* Are you reading something that is going to make a difference to your health or the health of your family? If it's not, then it probably isn't worth spending any of your energy on. I file things like that into the part of my brain marked "useless trivia for $200 Alex."

Unless you are one of those people who like to seek knowledge just for the sake of having it, you picked up my book because you were looking for something. Perhaps you have found yourself in the midst of your own health crisis. Maybe you have a spouse or other loved one who needs some nutritional help. Maybe you thought that this book contained the secret ingredient to dropping 20 pounds in 5 days while being able to eat nothing but cake and drink beer. (Sorry, that last one was in fact dripping with sarcasm.) No matter what brought you here, improving your health is worth your time and energy.

When I first began looking into changing my health, I was completely overwhelmed. I felt like I spent most of my time running in circles. I didn't know who or what to believe. Some experts were stating that meat was bad. Some would say that meat was good. We should or shouldn't eat grains and pasta. Fitness experts were both for and against running. It was confusing with a capital C.

I spent a great bit of time trying to decide who I would believe and who I would consider to be dishing out crap. In the end, I found that it came down to the three questions that I outlined in this chapter. Does it make sense? Is it true? And does it matter? Three simple questions to help you determine if the information is vital and worth your time. The rest is up to you.

Chapter 2

Get to know your food

There is no sincerer love than the love of food.
George Bernard Shaw

"Hello juicy Big Mac. How are you today? "

That is not exactly what I had in mind when I started this chapter. What I had in mind was learning more about where your food comes from, what exactly is in it and what happens once you put it into your body. All are important factors when making your food decisions.

The where?

How many of us really have an idea where our food comes from? I mean REALLY comes from? Aside from us walking into our local grocery store and selecting our dinner from the miles of shelves, have you put any thought into how the food gets from the farm/factory to your dinner table? How many people have a part in getting it there? How many ingredients are in it? What are all of those things on the label that you can't pronounce and where on earth did THOSE come from?

There is something to be said for eating fresh food from local suppliers. The biggest health benefit is that you don't usually wind up with food that has been pumped full of preservatives. If the supplier sells directly to the consumer, they don't have to worry about a long shelf life so naturally your food is fresher and contains less chemicals to keep it that way. Fresher food is healthier food. Right?

What exactly is a preservative anyway?

According to Merriam Webster: A preservative is a naturally occurring or synthetically produced substance that is added to products such as foods, pharmaceuticals, paints, biological samples, wood, etc. to prevent decomposition by microbial growth or by undesirable chemical changes.

Now, let's meet a couple of common preservatives that can be found in our food supply.

BHA or butylated hydroxyanisole is a commonly used preservative in food. It can be found in potato chips, instant mashed potatoes, preserved meat, beer, baked goods and dry drinks. It can also be found in rubber and petroleum products. BHA is highly used as a preservative because it is a high powered antioxidant. Do you know how anitoxidants protect food from spoiling? FAT.

Fats and oils in our foods have 3 long carbon chains. The more kinks in these chains, the healthier the fat. Unfortunately, when it comes to what makes a fat or oil rancid, the chemical bonds responsible for these kinks equate to a weakness in the fat's armor. Over time, oxygen in the air attacks the bond, which can transform the fat into a variety of chemicals, many of which smell foul and can be toxic.

When these fatty and oily foods are treated with BHA, the molecules occupy the attention of the attacking oxygen molecules and as a result, the food tastes better for a longer period of time.

BHA has been deemed by the Food and Drug Administration as "generally recognized as safe," while the National Institutes of Health says it's "reasonably anticipated to be a human carcinogen." In larger doses, BHA has been proven to cause cancer in laboratory rats. It was deemed "generally safe for humans" because the cancers that occurred in the lab rats occurred in an area of their stomach called the forestomach. Humans don't have a forestomach so therefore, it must be safe for our consumption. Right?

Next up? Sodium Benzoate. If you have ever taken a swig of soda and felt that slight tingle/burn in your throat, you have most likely consumed Sodium Benzoate. Sodium Benzoate is produced by a reaction of benzoic acid with sodium hydroxide, which makes it dissolve in water. The nice part about Sodium Benzoate? When mixed with Vitamin C, it forms an extremely carcinogenic compound. But no worries, the FDA has also deemed this one "relatively safe" for human consumption.

This JUNK, stuff like it and worse, is in our food supply. Again, repeat after me: Fresher is ALWAYS better.

Let's talk fruits and veggies for a minute so that we can further understand where our food is coming from.

Say that you and your friend want to enjoy some fresh orange juice and that you are lucky enough to have a shiny juicer sitting on your counter while your friend isn't as fortunate and must purchase packaged juice from the market. Here is the journey that your oranges typically take in order to become a lovely glass of orange juice for you to drink, depending on how you choose to get them:

Buying from the Supermarket

The oranges are grown at the grove.

They are usually sprayed &/or treated with pesticides and fertilizers.

They are harvested early, cleaned & treated chemically to remove the chemicals they were sprayed/treated with during growing.

The oranges are trucked to the manufacturing facility.

They are juiced.

The juice then has sugar, color ect added to make it appealing to Joe Customer.

The juice is then pasteurized to prevent spoilage. Pasteurizing = heating to kill any bacteria that it may have due to processing and to keep it squeaky clean when it gets dumped into its package. This is also the point that preservatives, vitamins, flavorings and any other added nutrients are added back to your "pure" orange juice because heating the juice to such high temperatures for pasteurization also cooks out just about every bit of nutrients. (And yes I said flavorings - as noted by Alissa Hamilton, with the Institute for Agriculture and Trade Policy and the author of "Squeezed: What You Don't Know About Orange Juice.")

The juice then makes its way to the packaging plant/area where it is packaged up and loaded onto pallets.

The pallets are loaded onto a truck for distribution.

The truck takes the pretty packaged juice to a storage warehouse where it will sit for sometimes months, before being distributed to various stores locally or to other transport means so it can be shipped worldwide.

The pretty packages are received in the stores

You, Joe Customer, buy that juice and take it home to enjoy.

**Total time from tree to your home:
30 days to many months**

Buying from a local grower

The oranges are grown at the grove.

They may be sprayed, depending on the grower.
They are harvested when they are ripe.

They are carried to the farmers market often as early as the same day they were harvested.

You purchase the oranges and take them home to juice up for your family.

Total time from tree to your home: 1 – 3 days

In plain English: buying local = fresher and healthier foods on our tables. Buying local usually translates into less chemicals in our food. Less chemicals in our food = lower risk of disease. Lower disease risk means less medications, less doctor visits and a healthier happier you.

What's In There?

I am frequently surprised by how many people buy and eat foods without bothering to read the food label. I am not talking about the calories either. What I am referring to is the most important part of your food label: the ingredient list.

On the food label you can find out how many calories your sausage biscuit has. You can see how many of the calories come from fat and whether or not that sodium level is something that you should be concerned with when you look at the label, but do you really know what is IN your food by reading only the nutritional information? Not really. To learn what is really in your food, you need to take a good hard look at the ingredient list.

Let's cozy up to THAT for a moment.

Nutrition Facts

Serving Size 1 Cookie (19g)
Servings Per Container 10

Amount Per Serving

Calories 90	Calories from Fat 30

	% Daily Value*
Total Fat 3.5g	5%
Saturated Fat 1g	5%
Trans Fat 0g	
Cholesterol 5mg	2%
Sodium 25mg	1%
Total Carbohydrate 13g	4%
Dietary Fiber 1g	4%
Sugars 9g	
Protein 1g	

Vitamin A 2%	•	Vitamin C 0%
Calcium 2%	•	Iron 2%

*Percent Daily Values are based on a 2,000 calorie diet. Your daily values may be higher or lower depending on your calorie needs:

		Calories:	2,000	2,500
Total Fat	Less than		65g	80g
Saturated Fat	Less than		20g	25g
Cholesterol	Less than		300mg	300mg
Sodium	Less than		2,400mg	2,400mg
Total Carbohydrate			300g	375g
Dietary Fiber			25g	30g

Calories per gram:
Fat 9 • Carbohydrate 4 • Protein 4

INGREDIENTS: SUGAR, ENRICHED FLOUR (WHEAT FLOUR, MALTED BARLEY FLOUR, NIACIN, IRON, THIAMINE MONONITRATE, RIBOFLAVIN, FOLIC ACID), ALMONDS, BUTTER (CREAM), NATURAL FLAVORS, BROWN RICE SYRUP, SALT, CINNAMON.

Contains Wheat, Almonds, Milk.

Check out the label next door. At the top is the nutritional information. Calories, Fat, Cholesterol, Sodium. All important information to know about your food however, if you take a look a bit further down the label, you will see the most important thing that you should pay attention to regarding your food: what is actually IN it.

The ingredients are listed according to percentage of quantity in each serving. On this label, you will notice that the first item listed is SUGAR. So each serving is made up of the large percentage of sugar.

My rule of thumb with the ingredient list is that if there are more than 5 ingredients listed, what you are about to consume is most likely a processed food.

Additionally, if one of those first five ingredients of that processed food is sugar in some format, you should make damn sure that what you are about to eat is worth the health ramifications it will cause you. And yes, sugary foods do cause health ramifications. (You can read more about that in the chapter 3.)

Another great rule regarding the ingredient list is to make sure you know what each ingredient is. If your diet is made up of processed foods, knowing the ingredients probably seems like a daunting task. (Who knows what Disodium Guanylate is anyway?) Here are some easy hints for you regarding deciphering labels:

- ✓ Ingredients ending in the letters "ose" are almost ALWAYS some form of sugar.
- ✓ Syrup in any format is sugar.
- ✓ Malts in any format are sugar.

It would be almost impossible to memorize the enormous list of ingredients that are used as preservatives, so I recommend that you stick to the list of common ones: citric acid, sulfur dioxide, ascorbic acid, propionic acid, nitrates and nitrites, sodium bisulfite, sulfites, and even formaldehyde. Preservatives allow the food to be stored/shelved for extended periods of time. Food that has been created to sit on a shelf for an extended period of time is NOT fresh.

BHT (Butylated Hydroxytoluene) is a highly toxic carcinogen that is used as a preservative in many foods, and should be avoided at all costs. It is used in jet fuels, rubber petroleum products, transformer oil and embalming fluid; according to it's material safety data sheet, it should not be allowed to enter the environment due to its impact on the aquatic environment and it's link to liver damage. And it can be found in our FOOD!

Yellow #5 and any other coloring should be avoided. Almost all colorants approved for use in food, are derived from coal tar and may contain up to 10ppm of lead and arsenic. Also, and not surprisingly, most coal tar colors could potentially cause cancer.

Propylene glycol alginate (E405): this food thickener, stabilizer, and emulsifier is derived from alginic acid esterified and combined with propylene glycol. Bear in mind that even though propylene glycol is used as a food additive, it has many industrial uses including automotive antifreezes and airport runway de-icers.

Are you scared yet? No need to be afraid of your food anymore. After you finish this book, you will be a warrior. Moving along...

Daily Values

Daily values are something that has been confusing people for a very long time. DVs were developed by the U.S. Food and Drug Administration (FDA) to help consumers determine the level of various nutrients in a standard serving of food in relation to their approximate requirement for it.

"Daily Value" is one of the fairly new terms used on food labels. It indicates the amount of a nutrient that is provided by a single serving of a food item. Daily Values are used to establish standards for comparison.

The Daily Value is actually based on two sets of standards. The first set of standards is called the Reference Daily Intake (formerly known as the U.S. Recommended Daily Allowance). It reflects the recommended level of intake for most vitamins and minerals.

The second set of standards, called the Daily Reference Values, is used for other nutrients that are also known to have a significant impact of health and disease. These other nutrients include fat, saturated fat, and cholesterol.

In plain English, you want the DV percentages for the icky items (saturated fats, sugars sodium and cholesterol) to be as low as possible and the nutrient rich parts (vitamins, minerals and proteins) to be as high as possible.

Simple enough to understand now, isn't it?

Organic, Low Fat & other labels

One of the most common mistakes that people make when looking at packaged food is being blinded by the shiny misleading words – organic, no/low fat, free range and all natural. I am in no way saying that labels lie, but, most of us are not fully aware of what exactly those words actually mean when you see them on a food label.

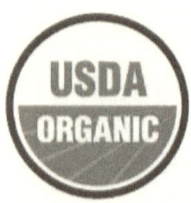 Let's look at the word "organic." It is usually packaged around the pretty green and white circle that the USDA likes to toss around but did you know that in order for a food product to wear that pretty green and white label, it is only required to come from 70% organic ingredients? Let me make this a bit more clear for you – just in case you are still confused – 30% of the ingredients in your organic processed food can be non-organic.

If you care enough to eat organic, then you should care enough to not buy processed foods that can still be made up of 30% garbage. Right?

How about the words "low fat" or my personal favorite: "fat free?" Eating a low fat diet is a great health choice however, it is important to understand that we do need to consume some fats in order to maintain our health. Just like some carbs are good for us and some are bad, the same rule applies to fats. (Carbs consumed from a baked potato, for instance, are ok for us to eat while carbs consumed via sugary soft drinks are not a good choice.)

Did you know that just about all candy is considered a fat free food? Instead of being loaded with fat, it is loaded with sugar and in most cases, chemicals. Fat free mayonnaise? It is indeed fat free however, it is loaded with sugar, artificial flavors and artificial preservatives. (aka: CHEMICALS)

This is why you need to concern yourself with the ingredient label first and foremost.

Some other labels you may see on your food:

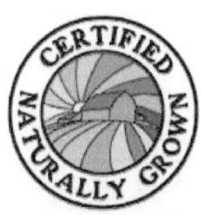

Certified Naturally Grown – Seeing this label means that your food was grown using the same standards as those for organic however, but the actual farm hasn't gone through the complete process to be certified by the USDA. Obtaining the "Organic" certification is expensive and time consuming so for some farms, especially the smaller ones, it's just not feasible. Having their food certified as Naturally Grown, lets you as a customer know that someone has certified that the food is indeed natural and that they haven't just slapped a word on the package in order to sell product.

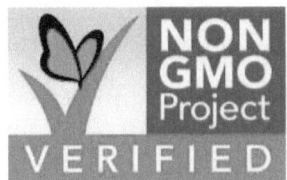

By now, just about every human on the planet has heard of GMO's. The non-gmo project is a non-profit group that provides a third-party labeling program in the United States for products grown without using genetic engineering of any sort - from seed to shelf. Please do not confuse THIS certification with a simple "Non-GMO" or "GMO Free." While companies can state that their products are GMO free, they are not tested and verified unless they are wearing the Non GMO Project label above.

Free Range – For poultry, this simply means that at some point in the day of the bird has been outside and that they don't "live" in a battery cage. It doesn't mean that the bird is fluttering around a meadow or spacious farm yard with a smile on it's little beak. The USDA doesn't currently have a legal definition for "free range" eggs nor ANY definition for "free range" beef or pork. So if you are looking at those items and they are wearing that label, they have simply slapped them on for sales purposes.

Let's recap:

- ✓ The best way to ensure that you aren't eating garbage is to eat FRESH foods
- ✓ Think about where your food comes from so that you can make an informed decision on whether to eat it or not.
- ✓ Don't eat chemicals disguised as food.
- ✓ Look first at your ingredient list, not at your calories/fat because the "WHAT" is more important than all of those confusing numbers.

✓ Understand the labels on a package and realize that sometimes, they are deceiving.

So now, take another look at your food. Really SEE it. Know where it comes from, what is in it, how it got from where ever it grew to your plate. Only then can you make an informed decision about what is going in to your body.

Chapter 3

Why you should stop eating crap.

Without health, life is not life; it is only a state of languor and suffering - an image of death.
Buddha

What exactly is health? If you are among the millions who surf the internet, you might believe that health is the absence of disease. The absence of disease? So if you don't have cancer, heart disease, diabetes or any of the other myriads of diseases out there, that qualifies you as healthy. Who believes that?

Health, as defined by Merriam Webster, is as follows: *The condition of being sound in body, mind, or spirit especially: freedom from physical disease or pain. The general condition of the body. A flourishing condition.*

Not just being free from disease but FLOURISHING.

How many of us have bodies that are flourishing? Do you feed your body foods that allow it to grow and rejuvenate itself? Do you drink enough clear liquids each day to ensure ample cell development? Do you exercise in a manner that strengthens your muscles and circulates your blood throughout your system?

I will go out on a limb and say that most of us don't.

Making the Connection

Do you know any human who will drive past a farm, look over at the peacefully grazing cattle and think "Wow, look at all of that steak?" Probably not the first thing that comes to mind when we see a grazing herd of cattle. Neither is the concern over whether or not those cattle have been eating hormone induced feed or whether or not they are being wormed and vaccinated.

Nor do we think about this herd when we are standing in the meat aisle at the grocery store getting ready to buy the burgers for this weekend's cook out. We just assume that because the meat is available to us in our store; that it's clean and safe. We also don't give much thought to the fact that about a month ago, it was once a living being who was peacefully chewing on some grass in the mid-west.

Why is it so hard to connect those two things? It is equally as difficult for most people to look at an orange tree and think about the process those oranges go through to get from that tree into our cartons of orange juice. As a society, we have been programmed to block all of that out of our brains. We don't HAVE to concern ourselves because we have these things readily available to us 24/7. It is a non-issue unless we head to our grocery store and the meat counter is empty – then suddenly we are learning all about mad cow disease and the finer details of the meat industry. Then, and only then, when our demand isn't being met, it's time to be concerned. Right?

Perhaps it's time that we wake up and realize that our food system is indeed in danger and that our health is already in crisis even though we may not yet feel or see our symptoms. Maybe we need to start THINKING about our food a bit more before we simply shovel it into our bodies like robots.

Were you aware that the growth hormones that they inject into cattle and pigs to make them grow at such an abnormal rate stay in the meat even after it has been processed? We are feeding those growth hormones to our family with each bite of that burger or bacon (Mmmmmm bacon...)

Do you think that it is such a trace amount that it doesn't matter because the FDA says it's no big deal? Take a look at this:

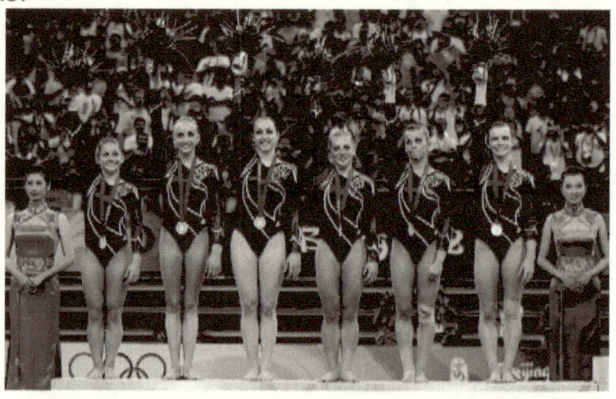

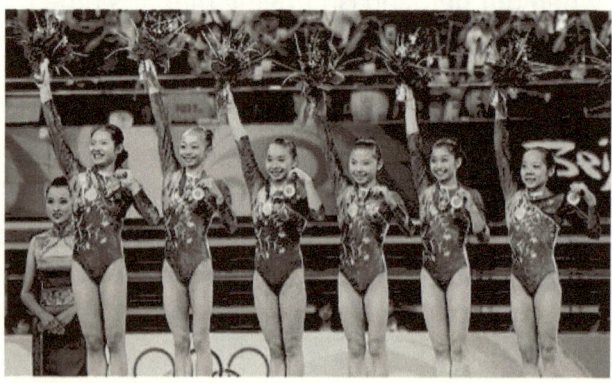

The photo on the top, is the US Women's Gymnastics team from 2008. On the bottom is the Chinese Women's team from that same year. Similar age spread, according to the Olympic Gymnastic   Committee (after the investigation into the accusations of China falsifying the age documents was concluded). So, what is the difference in these two teams? Why does the US team appear so much older than the Chinese team? Why do the US gymnasts have bodies of mature women while the Chinese team looks like young children? It's simple. Their diet.

The Standard American Diet (Humorously referred to by its acronym SAD) consists of meat, dairy, fruit, veggies and grains. In no particular order however, it is made up of a large quantity of meat and dairy. The Chinese standard diet consists of mostly grains, veggies and seafood. The Chinese rarely drink milk or eat cheese and their meat consumption consists mostly of fresh seafood, if any meat at all is eaten. Farm raised beef, pork and poultry is just not part of their diet.

Dr Tasnime Akbaraly, of the National Institute of Health and Medical Research in France conducted a study that was published in the American Journal of Medicine which clearly determined that the western diet (or standard American diet) greatly increased the risks of heart disease, diabetes and cancer as well as was a major contributing factor in premature aging. Dr. Akbaraly also concluded that avoidance of the "Western-type foods" might improve the possibility of achieving older ages free of chronic diseases.

Are you still sitting there thinking that the way that our beef is raised in the United States doesn't matter?

Let's reiterate to clear up any confusion: The Chinese diet is made up of mostly whole grains, veggies and seafood. Their slow aging process is noticeably visible even from a young age. They have a lower risk of cancers, diabetes, heart disease and other degenerative diseases. The average life expectancy of a Chinese citizen is 81 years. While the American diet is filled with hormone injected meats and dairy, fats, processed grains, artificially sweetened drinks, and chemically induced foods. Americans have the highest rate of cancers, heart disease, diabetes and other diseases over any other country in the world. The average life expectancy of a citizen of the United States is 76 years old.

There is no denying that diet does matter.

What can you do?

In 2007, after doing a crap ton of research, I decided to go completely plant based. For some people, making this much of a change is considered drastic. It was for me as well, but at the time, I was 120 pounds overweight. My father had heart disease. Several other relatives had cancer of some form or diabetes. It was time for me to do something drastic.

When I work with clients regarding making changes to their diets, I always ask them what they are willing to do for their own health. My number one recommendation for anyone that is seeking improved health is to begin transitioning to a plant based diet. Some will jump in with both feet and go completely plant based right off the bat. Some are scared to death to even consider reducing their pot per day coffee addiction let alone reducing their intake of McDonalds.

My rule of thumb is this: ANY positive changes you make will reduce your risks for developing disease. Therefore, we should not discount the small changes. There is not enough scientific evidence to support that you have to go 100% plant based with your diet in order to make improvements to your health, but it has been my experience that once you evaluate and start taking baby steps to improve your health, it won't take long until you are running full steam ahead.

My belief is simple. The more plants you can get into your diet, and the more animal products that you can remove from your diet, the healthier you will be. Please note that I didn't tell you that you had to join a cult and start making your own soap while munching on wheat grass to be healthy (but seriously, that would be amazing for your health.)
Here is what a plant based, whole food diet can do for you: (according to T. Colin Campbell in both The China Study and his latest book, Whole)

- ✓ Prevents 95% of ALL cancers including the types caused by environmental toxins.
- ✓ Prevents nearly ALL heart attacks and strokes.
- ✓ Reverses severe heart disease.
- ✓ Reverses type 2 diabetes.
- ✓ Reduces and eliminates inflammation in the body that directly contribute to arthritis and MS

In addition to doing this for your body, eating a plant based, whole foods diet can also do a lot for our environment.
- ✓ Significantly slows global warming.
- ✓ Reduces the need for deforestation.
- ✓ Reduces groundwater contamination.
- ✓ Ends the need for factory farms and their pollutants.
- ✓ Reduces malnutrition worldwide.

How can eating more plants help me to fight cancer?

We are going to get a bit scientific now. Don't wander off.

Our bodies are these amazing machines. We have been designed to perform some really awesome functions without even having knowledge of how to do them. We are born with a beating heart and functioning lungs and before we can even utter our first word our bodies are changing, growing and developing. Our cells multiply. Our blood carries nutrients and oxygen to our organs. We really are magnificent beings.

Keeping this in mind, think about the fact that we are all born with cancer cells in our bodies. Cancer doesn't fly into our bodies while we are outside running. We don't "catch" it from the grocery store cart. It is already in our bodies. Cancer, after all, is simply a cell that is growing at an abnormal and irregular rate.

So then, how do some people live their entire lives without cancer while others fight difficult battles with this disease?

Some cancers are directly caused by outside factors: cigarette smoking, alcohol use and environmental factors. Other cancers are related to infectious disease: Hepatitis B, HPV and HIV. However, according to the American Cancer Society, over one third of all cancers are directly connected to poor nutrition, obesity and physical inactivity.

I would like to go on record as stating that a very small percentage (less than 2% according to the ACS) of cancers are caused by direct genetic mutations. Genes do not determine disease on their own. Genes function only by being activated, or expressed, and nutrition plays a critical role in determining which genes, good and bad, are expressed. So, for all of you who sit back saying that you are genetically predisposed to lung or colon cancer because your Momma had it or your Grandpa had it – I call bullshit. You possibly have been raised on a specific diet, while living in a specific environment that will weaken your immune systems and permit cells in your colon to allow those cells to grow, but your Momma didn't make you get cancer any more than my dog made me get the flu.

Cancer cells abnormally grow in our bodies when our immune systems weaken and allow those cells to grow. If our immune system is strong, we lower our risk of developing cancer by over 75%. So then, how do we strengthen our immune systems?

When we eat plants, we are consuming copious amounts of antioxidants and phytochemicals. While animal products also contain antioxidants, the numbers are significantly higher by volume in plants. Animal products do NOT contain phytochemicals.

Antioxidants are vital to our immune health in that antioxidants attack free radicals. Radicals are the toxins that are in our bodies causing all sorts of damage to our healthy cells. Phytochemicals are the antioxidant helpers. I consider both of these guys vital to good health, don't you?

Plants contain vitamins and nutrients that are necessary for our body. More importantly, plant based foods are the ONLY foods that give us fiber. That's right, there is no fiber in that juicy T-bone, or in that cheese, those eggs, or the milk you drink. Slice it up, Buttercup. It's the truth.

So, if you want to significantly reduce your risk for all types of cancer, what should you do? That's right. Eat more plants and less critters.

What about Heart Disease?

Heart disease or atherosclerosis is caused from a build-up of cholesterol in the arteries. This build up leads to decreased blood flow and eventual blockage. If the blockage is not found, it leads to heart attack, stroke and heart damage.

Our bodies naturally produce cholesterol in our livers. We need it in our bodies in order to fuel our cells and function at tip top shape. We don't need large amounts of it, however. While plants do contain trace amounts of cholesterol in their cells, it is so miniscule of an amount that most science books neglect to mention it, leading some of the less curious to believe that plants don't have any of this lipid in their make up. When you consider that all animal cells have an abundance of cholesterol, it doesn't take long to come to the conclusion that eating animal products greatly increases the amount of cholesterol in our own bodies. One of the top ways to reduce the cholesterol in your body, according to the Mayo Clinic is to eat more fiber (IE: plants).

Certainly plants can't help with diabetes?

Diabetes is a disease that affects the way our body produces insulin. Insulin is produced in our pancreas and its purpose is to turn fats into glucose that can then be used for energy.

Each food that we put into our body has a level of glucose potential, and a group of lovely scientists have assigned foods a number on the "Glycemic Index" to give us a better idea of the amount of insulin our bodies will be required to have in order to process each food. (Have I confused you yet?)

Someone with type 2 diabetes doesn't produce enough insulin or their body is so screwed up that their body ignores the insulin, resulting in the glucose level in their blood being extremely high. Abnormally high levels of glucose in our blood can cause all sorts of ugly things to happen in our body. The short term effects of elevated glucose levels are feeling lethargic and weak, unsatisfied thirst, decreased immune system, blurry vision and frequent urination. The long term effects, if left untreated are much more severe. Kidney damage, heart disease, high cholesterol, and retinal damage resulting in blindness.

According to the Diabetes Association of America, the number one way to reduce the risk of and reverse Type 2 diabetes – Eat a low fat, high fiber diet. PLANTS!

An added note on diabetes: I have personally worked with several people who were diagnosed with either Type 2 diabetes or were at high risk for developing this disease. In all cases, these individuals adopted a plant based diet and have completely reversed this disease without the use of medications.

There are scientist, chemists and food professionals all across our globe who have far more experience than I do to recommend the benefits of shifting to a diet that is more plant based. The evidence of their research is readily available. If you are the type that likes to jump head first into that sort of thing, I highly recommend picking up a copy of The China Study or Dr. T. Collin Campbell's latest work – Whole. Both are very in depth studies of what I have reiterated here. (There are more works of reference listed in Chapter 10.)

Chapter 4

Don't Be a Pig

We eat as sons and daughters, as families, as communities, as generations, as nations, and increasingly as a globe. We can't stop our eating from radiating influence even if we want to.
Jonathan Safran Foer

Two Thirds of all American adults are obese. The obesity rates have more than doubled since 1980. We have an epidemic in the United States. If it continues, we will see an even higher rate of cancer, heart disease and diabetes, as these diseases are directly linked to obesity.

So, what gives? Why are we so fat? Let's do a little finger pointing, shall we?

Despite the rise in health care prices and the link between obesity and disease, the USDA has raised its recommended daily caloric intake by 30% over the past thirty years. It was 1800 calories per day in 1978. 2000 calories per day in 1990, 2300 calories per day in 2010. The fact is, our bodies need considerably less calories in order to function at a healthy level.

The number of fast food restaurants has more than quadrupled from 30,000 in 1970 to 140,000 in 1980. This number has been increasing at an equally alarming rate since 1980. Additionally, 90% of the money that we, as Americans spend on food is spent on processed food – food that comes from a box, can or package.

There was a trend in fast food around 2000. That is when you could order buckets of fries and everything could be Super Sized. As a society, we demanded more bang/fries for our buck. We gave no consideration to what these choices would eventually do to our health. All that mattered was that we got enough for our cash. In the mid 2000's, we all stood around in shock at how our neighbors were all huge in size and our family was dropping like flies from disease. Apparently, all of those fries also made us blind and stupid.

Thankfully, our trend has been shifting over the past five years. We are starting to wake up and understand that what we put into our bodies directly affects our health. We also are beginning to realize that if it took us a few years to pack on the extra pounds, that we can't expect to take a magic pill each morning while we still are not exercising and have those extra pounds fall off in a week.

It has always been entertained me to discuss the quantity of food we put into our bodies with people. Most have no clue what a portion is, let alone what it looks like on our plates. Hopefully, I can clear some of this up for you.

Portions are the measurement of food that the USDA uses to establish their recommended amounts to the American public. If you paid attention in Chapter 2, you already know where to find the portion information on a package label. That allows you to know how many calories and which nutrients each portion has in a particular food item.

You now know WHAT a portion is, but you may be wondering what exactly 8 ounces of spaghetti looks like. Here are some easy tricks to keep things simple:

- ✓ 8 ounces of protein is equal to the size of the palm of your hand (without your fingers) and approximately as thick as your index finger. Protein is to be considered as meat or legumes.
- ✓ A serving of bread is usually ONE slice or an individual piece.
- ✓ A serving of pasta is usually considered the amount of cooked pasta that will fit into one of those tiny, fancy tea cups. (I know. That is tiny.)
- ✓ A serving of fruit is usually the amount that you can hold in your hand without it falling. (One medium apple, a handful of grapes, etc)
- ✓ A serving of most beverages is eight ounces. On average, the diameter of the glass should fit into your palm (no fingers) and then measure up from the bottom of the glass up to the second knuckle of your thumb.
- ✓ A serving of veggies and grains (rice, quinoa, etc) is usually what you can cover with your hand if you leave your fingers flat and about an inch thick.

Now, what do you do with this brilliant information?

The next time that you put your plate in front of you, take a look at your portions. Really look at them. If you are trying to improve your health, you should have single servings of each group on your plate with the exception of veggies and grains. You can eat all of those that you want to...and you can do it without guilt.

After you have looked at your plate and can identify proper portions easily, you should try to make your plate as colorful as possible. The reason behind this is simple. Each "colorful" food on your plate usually brings with it a whole pile of nutrients that will improve your health. Nutrients from different colors of food do different things for your body. The more colorful your plate is, the more likely you are to meet the nutritional needs of your very amazing body in a healthy way.

If you happen to need to lose a few pounds (or a lot of pounds if that is the case for you) I highly recommend looking at your plate as if it were the face of a clock. Fill 2 hours of your plate with proteins or whole grains. Then fill the remaining portion of your plate with veggies and fruits. This is a simple trick to make at least 80% of your diet plant based and help you to reach optimal health.

But what about when I go out for a meal?

I use a very easy method for controlling my portions when I am at a restaurant. I order my meal and ask my wait person to bring a box when they deliver my meal. As soon as my food is in front of me, I place any excess into the to-go box and close the lid. It is very easy to dive into a delicious meal and lose track of all of the hard work you are trying accomplish. Next thing you know, you have devoured an entire plate full of rich pasta that was actually more like 8 servings rather than one or two. Don't even sniff your plate until you have your portions safely packed away and set aside. Then you can dive in and savor every last morsel that is on your plate.

Secondly, always order a vegetable with your meal and eat it first. I don't care if it's a side salad or a side of corn on the cob. Eat the veggie first. It will fill you up in a healthy way and keep your appetite in check. When ordering a salad, be sure that you order your dressing on the side rather than ON your salad. Dip your fork into the dressing and then stab your salad. This gives you the flavor with each bite without all of the extra calories that your salad swimming in ranch dressing would.

Lastly, if you order a drink when you sit down, wine, mixed drink or for crap's sake a SODA, be sure to drink water with your meal and don't refill the other beverage. My go to at a restaurant is iced tea. It's water and tea. Nothing more. I can drink it guilt free throughout my entire meal. It keeps my beverage intake where it should be without causing anyone to fuss over rules.

A few more rules on eating...

When you begin making changes to your diet, please remember that you have probably been eating this way for quite some time. You aren't depriving yourself of anything. You are merely changing the way you consume foods. If you really want a piece of the double chocolate lava cake, then by all means, you should have it. However, you should have a small piece of the not so healthy stuff rather than sitting down to eat an entire cake while watching True Blood.

Make sure that you SIT down to eat. Eating while multitasking is dangerous on several levels. You won't mindfully consume your meal if you are snarfing it down while driving to your next meeting. If you are pressed for time and find yourself in a rush when you get hungry, consider a healthy snack instead of a fast food meal being consumed from the front seat of your car. Carrot sticks and celery pack very well and will do wonders for your energy level while at work. Apples and other "to go" fruits have the same effect and are usually more difficult to gulp down.

Take time to eat. When you sit down for a meal, take a moment to appreciate it. Think about where it comes from. Admire how pretty it looks (because we know how to make our plates colorful now) and most of all, give yourself a pat on the back for fueling yourself with a nutritious meal. Meal time should be like a great date. Savor it; admire it; and remember that you don't want it to end.

And for crap's sake, put your fork down! This one simple act will slow down the rate in which you consume by over 50%. Slowing down how fast we eat keeps us from gobbling down air too, so we keep the post-dinner bodily functions to a minimum. Take a bite, put your fork down, and chew. Don't pick up your fork again until you have fully swallowed everything in your mouth. Your Momma will be so proud of your new found manners. I promise.

How is that for simple?

Chapter 5

Kick the Cravings

Chocolate is the first luxury. It has so many things wrapped up in it: deliciousness in the moment, childhood memories, and that grin-inducing feeling of getting a reward for being good.
Mariska Hargitay

"But I crave chocolate."

Cravings. They are some of my clients' biggest excuses for eating crap. While it is true that we have cravings, the process doesn't work exactly how we have been led to believe.

Hunger is triggered by a few different things. Most commonly, hunger is caused by a hormone released from our brain called leptin. Leptin is also responsible for letting your body know that is full. Hunger can be signaled by two stimulants: anandamide and neuropeptide. These can most commonly be found when they bind to canabanoid receptors – hellooo marijuana munchies.

While hunger is caused by a few different things, The result is the same: neurotransmitters in our brains trigger "feel good" moments for us as a result of the foods we eat. There currently is no scientific evidence that supports our bodies craving specific food. What we do crave are the chemical reactions that are caused by specific food items, not necessarily the food item itself.

Let me explain further.

When we divulge in eating sweets, the carbs kick start an increase in the level of insulin in our bodies. The insulin then clears out most of the amino acids in our blood stream. What we are left with is an amino acid called tryptophan. Most anyone who has eaten turkey on

Thanksgiving has heard of tryptophan. Tryptophan gets converted into serotonin in our brains, and serotonin makes us feel all warm and fuzzy inside. It has been proven that reduced serotonin levels are linked to depression. (Imagine if doctors could simply adjust the diets of the countless people who are currently taking anti- depressants rather than prescribing those people drugs?) With this information, we now understand that cravings are usually signals from our body that it wants the chemical reaction that we get from consuming certain foods.

I feel that cravings can also be habitual. Science may disagree with me but, I know that for myself, having something sweet in the evening before bed had absolutely nothing to do with any real need that my body had and instead, had everything to do with a very unhealthy habit that I had established. I had simply trained my brain that it needed to have a sweet before bedtime. This theory is evident not just with food either. Think about smokers. The nicotine is just one small part of the addiction and the habitual addiction is often the most difficult part of the habit to kick.

Now that we understand cravings a bit better, we are still faced with how to fight them off as we work to improve our health. When our bodies are sending us signals that we need something, we need to listen. Whether you are craving the chemical reaction to a food or you simply have a habitual need, cravings can very quickly derail your new lifestyle changes.

Ok, so, what should I do?

First and foremost, you need to take a step back and think about why you might be having these cravings. Identify whether the cravings are emotional or habitual. This isn't as complicated as it sounds. When you feel like you need to put something into your mouth, stop and count to ten. SLOWLY. Consider when you last ate food. If it was less than three hours ago, chances are you most likely have a habitual craving and not a real need for the food that you are about to eat. Put it back where it was and take a walk, do some stretching, or take the dog out for a game of fetch.

If your craving is in fact an emotional one, counting to ten will give you time to consider the choice that you are about to make. Is it indeed the healthiest one that you can make right now? Or are you simply trying to handle the need as quickly as possible? This will lead to binge eating or what I like to call "grazing". Grazing is when you try to satisfy a craving without really considering what it is that you need/want. You wind up consuming tons of other foods rather quickly without really listening to what your body is actually asking for. If you simply take a few minutes to listen to your bod, it will usually speak pretty clearly about what it needs and wants.

When our brain starts screaming at us to eat the food that we KNOW we shouldn't eat, there is only one thing to do: FIGHT BACK. If you had parents like mine, you know that the lesson to fighting well, is to outsmart your opponent. Right?

If you are transitioning from eating a diet full of processed foods and sweets, when you are sitting at your desk having a chocolate meltdown, how on earth do you expect to satisfy your brain's need for that creamy bit of pleasure? You give it chocolate of course. What? Did you think that I was going to tell you that you could never eat chocolate again? Fat chance. (pardon the pun) What you need to do is not deprive yourself of the things that you enjoy unless those things are going to cause direct harm to your body. Eating a piece of dark chocolate on occasion is NOT going to hurt you one bit. I promise.

Here are some of my favorite recommendations:

If you are a sweets eater, cut down your portions significantly. That way your brain isn't deprived but you aren't negating everything that you are working toward. It is a proven fact that as soon as our human minds think we aren't allowed to have something, that something is all that we can focus on. We aren't depriving ourselves, we are merely making healthier choices.

If it's a birthday, have a piece of cake, a small piece. OR a small scoop of ice cream. Enjoy every last morsel without guilt. Birthdays only come around once per year, after all. With cake, stick to the three-bite rule. Even if you are a ginormous pig, three bites will not cause you much grief. (Of course, NOT being a pig would allow you to keep holding your head high at the office parties and family reunions)

If chocolate is your passion, switch to a rich dark chocolate, NEVER EVER milk chocolate or white chocolate. Darker chocolate is packed with antioxidants so you can actually enjoy it without guilt. Lindt makes a great bar that can be found at most grocery stores. It is conveniently created into smaller squares. So when your brain is screaming for a chocolate fix, have a square of the yumminess. Savor it. Put the rest of the bar away for next time. It will keep safely for a long time in your fridge. Chocolate is awesome.

If you are a soda junkie, quit. Period. Soda is full of nothing but sugar, sugar substitutes and a chemical shit storm. There is absolutely NOTHING healthy about soda. And don't you dare sit there and think that you can't possibly give it up because I managed to kick an almost 200 ounce per day Pepsi habit without batting an eye. You just have to realize that what is in that can or bottle is KILLING you. Quitting that habit is much easier then. If it carbonation that you crave, switch to sparkling fruit juice. Make sure it is 100% juice and not some sugary juice crap pile, and only have one if you are on the verge of sporking someone in the eyes if you don't get a fizzy drink in your hand. You should never replace one bad habit with another.

Keep in mind that fruit contains natural sugars. If you aren't battling diabetes, and you feel like you need something sweet usually your brain can be satisfied with some yummy fruit instead of processed sugar crap food.

Think your brain is screaming for salty goodness? Try some crisp veggies with a bit of hummus or some fresh salsa. The veggies will give you the crunch without the crap and the hummus and salsa will satisfy that salty craving. (Writing that just made me giggle – I should write commercial jingles.)

Don't forget that seeds and nuts make AWESOME snacks. Find them in bulk and roast them yourself a few different ways, turning them into sweet treats, salty treats, or spicy treats. The great thing about seeds and nuts is that they are easy to pack up and take with you as well.

What if my cravings are habitual and not emotional?

This is an easy one. If you are staring at your life and realize that your craving is habitual – MAKE NEW HABITS.

When I needed to kick my nightly sweet habit, I simply turned it into something else: something better, something healthier. I was lucky enough to live in a home with a swimming pool in the back yard. So in the evenings, after dinner had been consumed and my kids got settled, when I normally would switch my thoughts over to the pint of Ben & Jerrys that I had stashed in the freezer, I began swimming.

Sometimes, I would do some laps. Sometimes I would just float around and stare at the stars. The most important thing that I did during this time though was to think about how great I was feeling instead of focusing on that Ben & Jerry's. It wasn't long until I tossed that freezer burnt carton out of my house.

A few notes on eating out of habit.

I was raised in the Midwest. While our household wasn't a farming household, most of our entire family was farm raised. Every single family event ever took place around a meal, sometimes more than one.

We had potluck picnics in the summer. A big sit down with all of the fixings at Thanksgiving. Breakfast AND dinner around the table at Christmas. Birthdays involving cake and food. Graduations. Births. Deaths. Everything was about food. Always. One of the hardest things that I had to do when making improvements to my health was to learn to eat when I was hungry rather than when it was lunchtime or "time for food".

I read a book in the midst of my research (I honestly forget which book it was) about finding your "hunger point". There was an entire chapter devoted to learning exactly what hunger was and how to recognize it in your own body so that you could eat when you were hungry.

I wound up going without food for three entire days in an effort to find my own hunger point. I did continue to drink water during these three days – I am not a complete bad ass. I know that sounds extreme but when you are 100+ pounds overweight, apparently you have a lot of excess fuel that your bod can use. Here is what I learned about myself during those three days:

• My stomach makes a lot of noise. Much of that noise happens right after I wake up and not because my body needs food.

• I will rarely hear my hunger signals but I always FEEL them. My belly just feels empty and I can actually feel that I am depleted of fuel.

• My mouth waters whenever I smell something delicious whether that be sweet smelling flowers, a juicy steak that I would never eat or fresh strawberries.

• I need much more liquid than I need food for my body to function happily.

• I thought I needed food much more than I actually did. Turns out that I am happiest with a cup of hot tea or coffee and bit of fruit in the mornings and then a bigger lunch and lighter dinner.

• Once I found my true hunger point, when my body actually said that it needed food, it was very easy for me to recognize.

It was more difficult for me to get out of the habit of eating at specific times than I ever thought it would be. Aren't we a funny society? My actual hunger point isn't dramatic or loud. It's not very ugly either. I do get a bit irritated if I push past my hunger point or if I work out until after I hit my wall; who doesn't get a bit fussy when they are hungry? In my body, my stomach just feels like it is empty and I can feel myself running out of energy. Sometimes, I will even get a bit shaky. I don't pass out. I don't collapse. I don't cry. If you try to get away with that crap, I will hunt you down and smack you. I promise. We are warriors who are taking control of our health, not pussy cry babies.

I encourage you to find your own hunger point. Snuggle up to it and learn what it feels like. If you are eating out of habit, stop. Emotional or habitual eating is what I imagine a really bad affair would be like. You know it's bad for you but until you grow some balls, you just go along with it because sometimes, it makes you feel ok. We aren't settling for ok anymore. Warriors conquer. Let go of the married, rich guy. You are a-ok to stand on your own two feet. I promise.

Chapter 6

Say I Love You – to you

Self-worth comes from one thing - thinking that you are worthy.
Wayne Dyer

One of the things that I absolutely love about yoga is that it forces you to turn your focus inward. When we are moving through asanas (poses, for you who have never been on a mat before) the focus isn't about sucking in our gut or flexing a bicep. We don't worry about what our hair looks like or if our manicure is chipped. The focus is on our breath and more importantly, our heart. Nothing else matters.

Yoga has indeed made me change my focus inward.

At one point, I was like most normal people. I would look in the mirror and instead of seeing laugh lines, I saw wrinkles. I saw chipped fingernails, frizzy hair and LOTS of jiggle. I had zero self-esteem and even less of a feeling of self-worth. I never would have put my bod on a yoga mat because "Oh my god, what would people think of me?"

Why do we do this to ourselves? Why has our society programmed us in such a way that we are more concerned with what people think and say about us than we are concerned with our own health and happiness? We have allowed the media to shove perfect looking celebrities in our faces and somehow they have made us feel like THAT is what we should strive for. Who set the bar for perfection?

There is a funny trend in the United States. We are so damn discontent. We don't like our jobs. We need better cars. Bigger houses. And...better bodies. I ask again, who sets the bar? Ladies, why is a size 5 THE perfect size to be? Men, why are you only "hot" if you have flowing locks and a 6 pack? I can tell you who sets the bar for our standards: we do. As consumers, we have let our entertainment, fashion, music and health industries lead us like sheep. We are to blame.

Why, then, do we make ourselves miserable trying to seek this drummed up idea of perfection? We look in the mirror and see stretch marks, muffin tops, wrinkles, gray hair, and decide that THAT isn't beautiful. The braver of us hop on a scale and if the numbers aren't in that perfect zone, we beat ourselves up because we aren't "perfect."

STOP IT. Just stop it.

Negative body image affects both men and women and it can lead to several not so nice things in our lives.
- ✓ Stagnant and unhealthy relationships: when you don't think you are worthy of great friendships or relationships, you don't exactly exude the qualities that people want to be around. People who lack confidence are also more susceptible to caving to pressure from others rather than making their own choices. You can begin to understand how this can have negative impacts on our connections with others.

- ✓ Lack of opportunities: often, a negative self-image makes it easier to doubt our abilities. When we aren't confident in our selves, we find it much more difficult to take risks, and then wind up missing out on things.
- ✓ Depression: need I say more on this subject? Happy, confident people do not suffer from depression.
- ✓ Poor health: negative body image has been linked to directly to obesity, eating disorders and drug & alcohol use not to mention increased stress levels. We all know what stress does to us. (heart disease, obesity, headaches, ulcers, high blood pressure)

It's time to realize that happiness comes from being able to look at yourself and accept right where you are. Today. It may not be the current version of perfection society is shoving down your throat but dammit, it's pretty great. Your heart is beating. You have the ability to move your body. More importantly, you have the ability to make choices. So it's time to suck it up Buttercup and let yourself off the hook a bit.

I am willing to bet that most of you who find yourself with this book in your hand are at least considering making some improvements to your health. (Some of you are reading just because you love me – THANK YOU.) Those of you who are considering changes, consider this for just one moment: what if, the next time you catch a reflection of yourself, you take a deep breath and just smile? Imagine how good it would feel to stop for two seconds of your crazy, hectic life and just think "I am going to be ok," or as my Momma would say, "I got this."

It changes your perspective a lot. It suddenly gives you some power, if even just for that brief moment.

If we can allow the bar to be set for us regarding what size house we should have, how many kids we should have, what type of car makes us cool – why can't we take that damn bar for everything else and put it wherever we want to?

I will let you in on a very important secret: we CAN.

When I first sat down to put my thoughts for this book into fruition, my only purpose was to empower people. To write enough of the right words that would give people permission to start thinking for themselves. To arm them with knowledge that they would feel comfy taking a hold of their reins. My vision for this book was also at one time, my own reality. I had a moment of looking at myself, all 250+ pounds of me and saying quite clearly "I am ok. Right now. Today. I am ok."

At the time, I didn't know much about food or my own body. I just know that I had taken the first steps to make positive lasting changes to my health and that no matter what happened yesterday or tomorrow, at that very moment, I was indeed ok.

I am a firm believer that we don't have much control in our lives. We can't change what people think of us. We can't change something from our past. We have absolutely no control over the moments in our future. We can only confidently be in charge of THIS moment. The one going on right now.

For most people, living in the present moment is a really difficult concept. It is largely in part due to what I mentioned earlier in this chapter. We are discontent. When we have this unhappiness in our lives, we spend all of our energy and time focused only on what is ahead of us, so much so that we let our "now" moments go flitting on by without a glance. We worry about things that we have absolutely zero control over, like "what-ifs."

The What If's.

What if I go to this party and they don't have anything healthy to eat? I may as well not even start because I go to a lot of parties. I will never be able to do this.

What if I have a bad day, go back to my old habits, and eat crappy? It is going to be hard. I should just give up now.

What if I can't find anything that I like to eat after I decide to make these changes? I will starve.

I know these things seem silly but they are all things that people have said to me while contemplating making improvements to their health. We have no way of predicting our future so why on earth worry about it? So, in answer to their questions, I always ask:

What if you succeed?

Think about that scenario. What if you find that you are really good at making healthier choices? What if it's easier than you imagine it to be? What if you find that you have an entire new pile of foods that you enjoy because you were brave enough to try? What if that day that you caught a glimpse of yourself in the window, and you smiled and thought to yourself "I got this" and you really believed it?

We can't let our what if's rule us into not even trying because as negative as they could be, they could also be positive. And what if?

Starting points

I am a list maker. I make them for everything; grocery lists, to do lists, goal lists. I love lists because they keep me focused. When I began my journey, I made another list: I called it my disaster list. It was a very temporary list for me. On it, I wrote down everything that I was worried about. EVERYTHING. My children being ill. My spouse dying. My dog falling into my pool. Hurricanes. My own health. Not being able to take care of my kids.

My list went on and on. I filled an entire legal page, front and back. I was apparently a worry wart. Once I had exhausted my brain trying to list every little thing that I was worried about, I picked up a red ink pen. I began going back over my list and marking off everything that I could do absolutely nothing about. Do you know what I was left with? I had one single thing left on my list. The one thing that I felt like I had some control over right that second: my health.

It was quite a shocking realization for me. I bet that if you sat down right now and made your own disaster list that you would wind up at the same darn reality check as well. The only thing that we can have control of right now, in this moment is our health.

Now What?

You know how that old saying goes: you can't expect to get different results if you keep doing the same thing that you always do. At some point, we have to decide to take a first step toward change. Maybe your first step was reading this book. Let's make the next step realizing that you are the one in charge of your health, your life and your own happiness. Not your spouse, your parents, your kids or your friends. YOU.

Most of us forget to consider our self-worth. We don't think it's appropriate to pat our own backs so we are left with standing around waiting for others to toss us a bone and give us that kind of appreciation. What happens when the people that we have no control over forget us? Or don't have us at the top of their priority lists? We wind up being unhappy and sometimes even angry. Guess what Health Warrior? YOU can pat your own back. Love yourself. Don't wait for someone else to.

Here is what I mean:

Scenario: a stay at home mom of two small kids is married to a very hard working hubby. Hubby gets up each day before the sun comes up and goes to his job. He works hard for a boss who is quite an asshat but pays hubby well enough that stay at home mom can be what she has always dreamed of being – a SAHM. Hard working hubby often works late and comes home tired. While SAHM runs the house like a well oiled machine, she sometimes feels like hard working hubby doesn't notice the shiny mopped floors and doesn't understand the effort she puts in to prepare the gourmet dinners each night. She too is often tired when hard working hubby comes home. Both parties work hard. Both feel under appreciated. Both think that the other should be doing more for their marriage and to make the other feel better. This leads to bitter feelings. The SAHM mom yells at hard working hubby because he never brings her flowers or makes comments about the gourmet dinners. Hard working hubby yells because SAHM is always adding to his stress by pointing out where he is lacking when all he has ever done was work really hard so she can stay at home with the kids.

Now, imagine if SAHM took a step back. That she looked at her children and her beautiful home and found a sense of pride in keeping that home looking beautiful and those kids happy. What if she didn't rely on hard working husband for her flower fix and instead bought her own flowers when she felt like she could use some added brightness in her day. What if SAHM took a few moments at dinner time and excitedly shared with hard working hubby how happy it made her to find this great new recipe for the delicious meal she whipped up tonight and also told him how much she appreciated him working so hard so that she had time to follow her passion of gourmet cooking.

SAHM took control of her own happiness. She patted her own back when she needed it. She doesn't come across as selfish. She comes across as happy and healthy. She isn't lacking one damn thing because she LOVES herself. She wakes up in the mornings, looks at herself in the mirror and says "I got this."

Give yourself permission to look in that mirror each morning and say "I Got This" and then give yourself permission to believe it. We have to start somewhere. Pat your own back. Love yourself. Baby steps can lead to a really amazing journey.

Chapter 7

Move Your Ass

Exercise is done against one's wishes and maintained only because the alternative is worse.
George A. Sheehan

You would think as a personal trainer, running coach and yoga instructor that I would find it quite easy to write about exercise, but the fact is that there is NOTHING about exercise that is easy. You sweat. You breathe heavy. Your muscles ache. I personally have a love/hate relationship with exercise and depending on my weather in South Florida, sometimes the heat and bugs make me hate exercise a lot.

When I work with clients, they are often surprised when we begin analyzing their exercise routines. Many people think that when I recommend that they move their bodies that I am only talking about running for miles, lifting hundreds of pounds of weights, or anything else they do in a gym. While all of those things are indeed considered exercise, there is so much more for us to consider when we are counting up the ways we move our bodies, and most of these things fall nicely into the definition of exercise, so we shouldn't discount them.

Exercise is considered any activity requiring physical effort, carried out with the intent to sustain or improve health and fitness. Considering this, can we then put our daily jaunts up the office stairs in the exercise category? How about our trudge through the grocery store? Or the walk that we take with our dog every night? YES WE CAN.

Since every body is indeed different, each person will have different needs and will respond differently to certain types of exercise. I always recommend that if you have not been exercising regularly, that you don't just jump in and expect to be competing in an ironman event a month from now. Just like with our diets, I believe in the baby step theory. We start small and gradually add on as our body adjusts to it's new found routines. You are not required to join a gym or run out and fill your home with expensive exercise equipment. I like to keep things more simple than that. Plus, if you get into the habit of exercising on equipment either at home or at a gym, what happens when you travel? Let's make habits that we can stick with – no matter what.

Where do I begin?

Our bodies are designed to see a vast improvement to our health with only ten minutes of cardio work each day. If you are severely overweight or you have underlying conditions such as heart disease or diabetes, ten minutes each day will be a great starting point for you. Ideally, of course, you would plan for a more vigorous routine in your near future.

When you start to evaluate your lifestyle, I recommend that you be honest with yourself. Don't put swimming on your list of possibilities if you hate the water because you most likely won't stick with it. If you hate bugs, don't plan for a heavy list of outdoor activities. Don't just focus on one particular activity either. Different movements work different muscles in your body. Additionally, different activities will keep you from getting bored stiff. The main thing is that you don't overextend your body, your finances, or your abilities with whatever you choose to pursue. Those are sure fire ways to set yourself up for failure.

WHAT do I start with?

Exercise, when we first start out, SUCKS! It really does. While we may have a sense of feeling like we are moving forward because we have finally jumped in to do something to improve our health, it is still hard. The best thing that I have found is to find the types of exercises that you are really interested in. If you have always wanted to learn to play tennis, utilize that to get your move on. Learn to wakeboard, snow ski, join an adult swimming club, try out the hot new salsa club in town...you get the idea.

At the top of my recommendation list is walking. I also recommend that you have a plan to slowly transition into becoming a runner. The main reason that I have a love for running is that you begin by walking. EVERYONE can walk. It doesn't matter what you think your physical limitations are, or if you have been injured in the past; you can walk or run anywhere, anytime, and with anyone. You don't need any equipment so it is hard to find excuses to not do it. It's also really inexpensive and highly effective; in other words: SIMPLE. With three teenagers, a husband that I like to keep happy and half a zoo full of critters to tend to, I LOVE simple.

The Starting Line:

I have a couple of very simple rules when it comes to beginning a walking program. The first is that you have to walk. You don't stroll. You don't meander. You walk like you have a purpose. That purpose is to improve your health. It is ok to take your dog along, as long as he or she will allow you to keep him or her on task and not require you to stop at every mailbox. Take your kids. Your spouse. Your neighbor. Just be sure to let any walking partner know that you are walking for exercise and that your health depends on it and don't let anything deter you from that.

I don't like to mess with checking heart rates or respirations so I use the talking/singing guide, or as we coaches like to call this, the level of exertion scale. Quite simply, level 1 you are just waking up, you aren't moving your body – things are as easy as they can be. At level 10, you are falling over gasping for breath and you are contemplating your mortality. Understand? With that in mind, when you begin your program, you walk at a pace that allows you to talk however you should have difficulty trying to sing. This places you very nicely on the level 3 side of that scale. Walk with purpose.

Secondly, you have to walk with a smile on your face. I know that is a strange request, but you need to feel good about improving your health. You are doing what you need to do. You are willing to get hot and sweaty or freeze your ass off in order to reach your goals. You are reducing your stress levels, lowering your blood pressure, reducing your cholesterol, and helping to improve your sleeping patterns. THIS should make you giddy. When things make us giddy, we smile. Remember that famous line from Reese Witherspoon in Legally Blonde: "Happy people don't kill their husbands." (or their kids or their neighbors – you get the idea.)

I recommend that you walk every OTHER day. This gives your body and your mind a day to rest and recover. No matter how gung ho you are to jump in with both feet, rest days are imperative to your health. Rest days allow your muscles time to rest in between workouts. They allow your immune system time to recover from the added stresses of workouts and more importantly, rest days give your mind a day off.

When you first begin your walking program, plan to purposefully walk for twenty minutes. Remember that purposeful walking is a pace that allows us to talk but not sing easily. Strolling for a few minutes to let your body get into exercise mode and warm up before you begin. Your warm up also helps you turn your focus to your workout before you jump right in. Add a five minute "cool down" at the end of your purposeful walk and you now have added thirty minutes of exercise to your healthy routine.

The Wicked Warrior walking plan:

- ✓ every OTHER day
- ✓ 5 minute warm up walk

- ✓ 20 minutes at a pace that makes it difficult to sing but not to talk
- ✓ 5 minute cool down

Transition to running:

Since I was active as a kid, I had tried just about everything that I had ever wanted to. Competitive swimming, tennis, martial arts, snow skiing. What was on my bucket list as an adult was to run a half marathon. I know to some, this doesn't seem like a huge challenge but when you factor in that I had severe asthma as a child and I have always struggled with breathing efficiently, running 13.1 miles just seemed to be a super hero type of thing for me and exactly what I needed to motivate myself to keep moving when I was 100+ pounds overweight.

Most people that turn to running have either run in the past and want to pick it back up again, or they have no clue what they are in for and merely want to complete a race for the bragging rights. I admit, when I first decided to hit the pavement, it really was just for bragging rights.

When you are completing your walks and are getting bored stiff in the middle, it's time to add a pep to your step and call yourself a runner. Don't be scared. Running scares the shit out of most people. Most have heard horror stories or had a bad experience themselves. But making the leap into the world of running is actually full of really amazing things. Running is by far one of the most efficient forms of cardiovascular exercise there is. So it shouldn't be so damn scary. Right?

My number one recommendation for transitioning from a walker into a runner is to take off your shoes. Yes. You read correctly. Take off your shoes. When you run barefoot, you will run lighter. You will connect with the energy of the earth and it will be far more difficult to ignore the cues that your body will be sending you along the way.

Let's tackle some of the fears that people have expressed to me when I suggest barefoot running to them.

What about glass, rocks and worse yet hypodermic needles? I don't know about you but I live in Miami. A big city. Tons of people around. Lots of traffic. Tourists. I have been running barefoot for over 2 years now and I have encountered glass one time during my run. I have yet to encounter a needle. I run mainly on sidewalks. The last time I checked, most people usually look where they are going when walking and running. It is easy to spot debris in your path and simply run around it. I have ever only had one "wound" from a run. I managed to find a thorn from a shrub. It took me two steps to feel it, stop and extract it from my foot, and then proceed with my run.

Aren't you worried about athlete's foot or other diseases? This one always makes me laugh. Athlete's foot is a fungus. It thrives in dark, moist environments. How dark and moist are your feet when you have your shoes off? It is actually HEALTHIER to have your feet out of your shoes than in them. If I happen to have any scratches, blisters or any other open-type injuries on my feet, I wear my Vibram shoes. It's not rocket science.

It's not good to run without the support of shoes. Really? Tell that to your 5 year old. We have been programmed to think that we need expensive running shoes when in fact, all that these shoes do is keep us slaves to the shoe industry. Bunions, hammer toe, and muscle weakness are all caused from shoes. You run without shoes and your feet do the job they were designed to do. They support you. Repeat after me: You don't need shoes, you need stronger feet.

I can't run. My hips and back always hurt when I try. Do me a favor, put on your favorite sneakers and stand up in them. Feel how high your heel is off of the ground. If you are in a standard running shoe of this season, you are probably standing with your heel elevated about 1 ½ - 2 inches from the floor and your heel is also about an inch higher than the front of your foot. Now, take your shoes off and place your foot on the floor. Stand up. Now, pick your heels up about an inch from the floor. What does that do to your balance? How does it feel in your hips and lower back? Are we beginning to see a point here?

When our heel gets elevated above our forefoot, it requires us to shift our entire body backwards in order to keep from falling over. It puts a sway in our lower back and added stress on our hips. Now, imagine this added stress being jarred, repeatedly for a mile or two. Do you understand why running shoes can sometimes be the cause of our running issues? No matter how squishy and cloud-like they feel, if they force your alignment off, even just slightly, they can cause you issues.

There are tons of reasons why I like to run barefoot. For me, it just makes sense and seems to really work for my body. While I don't run barefoot all of the time, it sure helps to tackle any issues that arise before they lead to injury.

So, you have moved on from walking to having the need to run. I have convinced you (sort of) to start off bare footed. Now what?

You already have your base workout under control. You currently walk every other day. You have a 5 minute warm up to get your head in the game so to speak, you walk with purpose for 20 minutes and then you have a 5 minute cool down. All you need to do now is add in some running intervals.

Intervals are great for building up stamina. All that you really need is a watch with a second hand or a smart phone with an interval app. When we move to jogging instead of just walking, you will move up that level of exertion chart to a 5. (Remember that 1 is lying in bed first thing in the morning while 10 is what you would be like if you were keeling over and having a heart attack) We want to be working right in the middle of those two while we are running. In the running world, this is our long run pace. You can stay working at this level for a decent amount of time. You should still be able to talk at this pace.

Remember the baby steps that I mentioned earlier? They come into play here as well. We begin with a nice set of easy intervals and will slowly add on to them each week until we are running a distance that makes us happy. Easy as pie.

The Wicked Warrior running plan:
- ✓ Week 1: 5 minute warm up then alternate the following: 60 second jog followed by 90 second walk. Repeat for 20 minutes. 5 minute cool down.
- ✓ Week 2: 5 minute warm up. Alternate 90 second jog followed by 2 minute walk. Repeat for 20 minutes. 5 minute cool down.
- ✓ Week 3: 5 minute warm up. Alternate 2 minute jog followed by a 2 minute walk. Repeat for 20 minutes. 5 minute cool down walk.
- ✓ Week 4: 5 minute warm up. Alternate 4 minute jog followed by 2 minute walk. Repeat for 20 minutes. 5 minute cool down.

- ✓ Week 5: 5 minute warm up. 5 minute jog, 3 minute walk, 5 minute jog, 3 minute walk, 5 minute jog. 5 minute cool down.
- ✓ Week 6: 5 minute warm up. 8 minute jog. 4 minute walk. 8 minute jog. 5 minute cool down.
- ✓ Week 7: 5 minute warm up. 10 minute jog. 3 minute walk. 10 minute jog. 5 minute cool down.
- ✓ Week 8: 5 minute warm up. 25 minute jog. 5 minute cool down.

At this point, you can begin measuring your runs in distance. 8 weeks in should have you running close to 2.5 miles. WOW, I bet you never thought that would happen, did you? Congratulations. You are a runner.

My love for yoga

I simply can not write this section of this book without discussing yoga. It is by far my favorite way to move my body as well as one of my favorite things to share with others. I came to yoga about half way through my journey to health and really had no clue what it would do for my body or my mind; I just knew that at the time, all of the cool kids were boasting about yoga classes. So I had to check it out.

Yoga is not exercise. It is a discipline. While you may dunk your toes into yoga for the benefits that the poses bring to your body, even the most close-minded individual will quickly feel all that yoga is.

Yoga is an ancient practice of breathing, meditation and asanas. It is practiced for improving health, relaxation and managing your stress levels. Yoga is a union of your body and your mind.

I hope that all of this spiritual talk isn't scaring anyone off.

In plain English, yoga is a series of "poses" that when combined with specific breathing techniques, will improve your balance, your strength and will indeed lower your stress levels without the typical physical stress that many forms of exercise can put on your joints. With those things alone it is worth it's weight in gold as far as exercise goes. What makes yoga so dynamic is that when you are moving through these asanas, you are engaging even the smallest of your muscles. So an hour on your mat works out every inch of your body. That is hard to come by when you are trying to find sufficient ways to work out.

Yoga typically gets discounted by the die-hard toughies as not being a "real" work out however, it has been my experience that the people who discount yoga have never really practiced yoga.

While moving through the asanas, you use guided or "conscious" breathing. Filling your lungs to capacity and then releasing your breath with just as much thought. This type of conscious breathing has HUGE benefits on our health.

- ✓ From a physical standpoint, we have to have oxygen or we die. Oxygen feeds our cells and while most people think that if they are breathing in an out they are healthy, the truth is that most of us do not get enough oxygen to promote optimal health through our normal breathing.
- ✓ There has been much research showing that by altering our breath patterns, we can change our mental and emotional states. We are capable of changing our own chemistry and mental states simply by performing conscious breathing.
- ✓ Most of the toxins that are in our bodies are released through our breath. Upwards of 70%. Imagine, then, consciously breathing in full breaths of oxygen and releasing all of the toxin-filled carbon dioxide from your own body with EVERY SINGLE BREATH that you exhale.
- ✓ Deep, full breathing works to massage your internal organs. How great do your muscles feel after a good massage? Isn't it cool that we can do the same for our kidneys, liver, pancreas, heart and lungs? Take a breath and massage away.
- ✓ Do you suffer from high stress, anxiety, or hyper tension? Sit and breathe consciously for a few minutes. It really does lower your heart rate, blood pressure, and stress level.
- ✓ By consciously breathing, we retrain our diaphragm. It allows us to breathe more freely in all situations, as well as increasing our lung capacity.

Now, add the benefits of the conscious breathing to the benefits of each of the asanas:

- ✓ Improved balance. As we practice yoga, we become very aware of our own bodies. Each asana is designed so that as we turn our focus inward, we FEEL different parts of our own bodies. This helps us to feel more confident with our physical selves, making it far easier to keep ourselves in balance physically and emotionally.
- ✓ Improved flexibility. This is a no brainer to me. Flexibility is imperative to joint support and mobility. Flexible bodies are happy bodies.
- ✓ Improved body awareness. Body awareness is probably the main reason that I recommend yoga to every person that I come in contact with. Having body awareness puts us in touch with ourselves physically but also emotionally. It is difficult to be unhappy and depressed when we can actually FEEL our bodies on the inside.
- ✓ Improved immunity. Yoga promotes maximum oxygen intake with the least amount of stress on our bodies. Healthy cells make for healthy bodies.

It begins to become apparent why I love yoga so much. Combine a regular yoga practice with regular cardio exercise and you are destined for great health.

There are many options for practicing yoga. I highly recommend that for your first experience with yoga, you attend a guided practice. I don't care how super hero like you are, you will NEED and benefit from the modifications that a trainer instructor can give you in a class. Once you are comfortable with the breathing techniques and the basic asanas, it will be safe for you to practice at home as well.

Guided classes are great ways to push yourself a bit further SAFELY as well as surrounding yourself with amazingly positive people. Most studios will offer drop-in rates that allow you to come try out a class or instructor without any type of contract. Go get bendy.

*I have also included some great web sites and smart phone apps that get the Wicked stamp of approval in the last chapter of this book so that when you are ready, you are loaded up with everything you need to be your own yoga addict.

Chapter 8

Keep It Simple

If we could give every individual the right amount of nourishment and exercise, not too little and not too much, we would have found the safest way to health.
Hippocrates

I contemplated naming this my cheerleading chapter because that is what it comes across like to me when I read all of my notes. Really though, it is more about sharing my best advice to anyone who is staring at a list of things that they need or want to change about their health: Keep It Simple.

I love food. I have always been very honest about that. When I made the changes in my life, the last thing that I wanted to do was to spend time counting and adding up calories. Nor did I want to spend hours hunting down weird ingredients that I had never heard of before to make food that took hours to prepare. I have much better things to do with my time. I am going to share with you what I did to keep myself sane as I began transitioning to a healthier life.

Throw away your fricken scale.

A scale is a way to measure progress when we are trying to lose weight. Why then am I telling you to toss it? Because you aren't trying to lose weight, you are trying to live your entire life in a healthier manner. If your body has pounds to drop, it will drop them without you having to step on the scale every damn day. Stop trying to use numbers to evaluate your health.

We are obsessed with our scales and being at an ideal number, when reality is that we are all built differently. We have different body compositions, different bone densities, different metabolisms, different base caloric needs, so why on earth would we try to pigeon hole our measure for success?

Put your scale in a closet and start paying attention to how you FEEL. If you are feeling bloated and tired, you aren't eating properly. Change what you are doing. We get so hung up on numbers, that we start doing desperate things to get those numbers to say what we think we want them to say. We quit listening to our own bodies. Hide your scale and start paying attention. You will be much happier.

Don't count calories.

I can not stress this enough. Do you REALLY want to be sitting at the table of a fancy restaurant with your significant other sitting across from you while you pull out your smart phone app to tell you if you should order dressing for your salad? Follow the few rules you have to follow and eat the foods that make you happy and healthy. Rule reminders:
1.) Don't eat food that comes from a box.
2.) Fill 80% of your plate with plant based foods.
3.) Don't be a pig and don't overeat.

If you are eating plant based foods, you will eat the right type of calories, so quit obsessing about it.

Change your attitude.

It is a known fact that as humans, we are programmed to want the things that we can't have. If you go into these health changes looking at them as a temporary change, that is what your health will be: temporary. Don't convince yourself that you can no longer have chocolate or a piece of Aunt Tilly's birthday cake, because deprivation is the quickest route to failure. YOU are in charge and you know how to make the right choices. This is no longer about the CAN'T. You CAN and you WILL.

Don't be afraid to ask.

I am talking about your choices. No matter what situation you are in, you have them. You aren't "stuck" with whatever is on the menu at a restaurant. Going out for a meal after I made my dietary changes always seemed to be a bigger deal to my family than it ever was for me. I always knew that I could order a salad - no matter where we went - so anything I could find beyond a side salad fell within my new eating habits was a huge bonus. Attacking a menu, charming a busy server and enjoying a lovely meal out was always an amazing adventure to me, and that is exactly how I approached it every single time. Let me say that I have eaten at burger joints, barbeque places, and even at a steak house...without any hostile situations being encountered.

My trick: smile and ALWAYS be polite, no matter what weird stares you are met with. Most places are quickly learning to accommodate their healthier clientele. I recently had one of the best meals of my life after having a friendly conversation with our server about my diet. She got especially excited when I told her there were no veggies that I didn't like and gave her and the chef free reign to whip something up.

A couple of notes when ordering out:
1.   You can almost always order pasta dishes and salads sans meat if you ask.
2.   Don't be afraid to ask your server for suggestions when ordering.
3.   Be adventurous and open to trying new things. Our taste buds change every 30 days. Something that you didn't like as a kid might quickly find itself on your list of favorites as a healthy eating adult.

You are different.

You aren't your brother, your mom, or your best friend. You are YOU. You have your own set of needs, your own thoughts and your own way of doing things. Your own likes and dislikes. Recognize that. Embrace it. If we were all exactly alike, wouldn't this be a boring little world? Be ok with being you, period.

Don't rely on others to make you healthy.

If there is one message that you have picked up from this book, I hope it is that you are the one ultimately in charge of your own health. YOU. You know that you need to eat differently. You know that you need to move your body. Stop depending on your friend to show up before you go out for your run. Spend time with your favorite person on the planet: YOU. You don't need a cheerleader. You don't need anyone to hold your hand. Some of my best thinking happens on my runs. I am out there alone and have nothing to do other than listen to my own body…and my thoughts. While at first it freaked me the hell out, I have really begun to enjoy being able to be in my own head for a little while each day. It has taught me that I can indeed stand on my own two feet, and while I appreciate the cheerleaders in my life, I don't NEED them to move forward. They are simply my added bonus.

Take photos of yourself.

Yes, I said it. Keep in mind that I was 100+ pounds overweight when I started. I still stood on my pool deck while my sweet daughter snapped a photo of me. I recall looking at that photo the day it was taken and crying. I was so sad and unhappy that I allowed myself to get to that point, but that photo also marked a HUGE turning point for my life. THAT was the day that I took control of my own health.

I have continued to take full body selfies, about every 6 months. It's not an ego thing – TRUST me. I simply recognize that there are days when I will need a reminder of where I came from and where I am headed. The photos also allow me to easily see my progress, which isn't always easy to do when we are traversing along towards health.

So, no matter how difficult it may be, look right into that camera lens with the eyes of a health warrior and take that photo. You won't regret it.

Surround yourself.

There is no better way to stay focused on your health than to be around people who are focused on their health. People who are focused on their health will eat better. They will discuss exercise. They will share inspiring stories. They WILL BE HAPPY.

When I began making changes to my own life, I quickly realized that few in my circles were very health based so I had to really seek out healthy influences.
The first stop on my to-do list was joining an organic produce buying group. This not only gave me an excellent source for TONS of yummy produce, it also put me face to face with people who had TONS of recipes, hints, and tricks for eating better. These people shared information about healthy activities when they got together. They shared the different ways that they got their own kids to eat better. They shared locations of great restaurants in my area. The knowledge that appeared at my fingertips through this circle was abundant.

Another great resource for surrounding yourself with all things healthy is the internet. I sought out blogs and web sites, signed up for mailing lists, and started hunting down some great recipes to try. It didn't take me long to expand my circle of healthy, happy people. (A list of some of my favorites is printed in the last chapter of this book.)

Don't be afraid.

Change can sometimes be scary, especially if we don't have a clear idea of where we are heading. This is definitely NOT one of those scary piles of change. This is one of the happiest adventures of your life.
Get out and try new activities. Try new foods. Meet new people. What have you got to lose?

Don't stress.

One of the biggest mistakes that people make is to go at change with an all or nothing attitude and expect to be perfect from the very beginning. There are very few of us who are true super heroes. We are, however, all human. We have bad days and we make mistakes. So be prepared to cut yourself some slack, and don't be quick to just throw in the towel.

I like to look at each choice we make as an individual event. If you get up in the morning and wolf down a not-so-healthy breakfast, is it really the end of the world? Or merely one single bad choice? As our day progresses, we have two more meals and probably a couple of snacks to do right. Correct? So don't beat yourself up for that ONE slip. Acknowledge it, let it go, and move along.

A bit more on stress.

Stress is the body's reaction to situations that requires adjustment or change. Some stress is actually good for us in that it keeps us alert and away from bad situations, of course, stress, without relief can result in some very bad health implications such as headaches, trouble sleeping, digestive issues, high blood pressure, heart related issues, and even promoting the growth of cancer cells.

These health issues arise when our bodies have too much cortisol in our system. Cortisol is the chemical that our body produces when exposed to stressful situations. A bit of it is good for us, lots of it is bad. The key is to find a healthy balance. Easier said than done for most normal humans.

In managing stress, most of us bring a lot of our challenges on ourselves. We tend to worry and dwell on things that we have absolutely no control over. I have found that when I find myself being a worry wart, asking myself three simple questions helps find a solution to deal with the stress.
   ✓ *Is this situation directly affecting me or my family?* If it isn't directly affecting you, LET IT GO.

If it is affecting you directly, work to find a solution.

- ✓ *Is this situation something that I can do anything about right now?* If you have control, then you have an opportunity to fix whatever is wrong. If it isn't something you can do anything about right now, let it go until you CAN do something.
- ✓ *Does this really matter?* Often, in the heat of a moment, we are fueled by emotions. Emotions can make us feel passionate about something that in ten minutes' time, we won't feel so passionate about. If you give yourself a few minutes to think before you act, it can keep you from acting irrationally and possibly causing more stress and chaos in your life.

No matter how we look at it, we live in a stress filled world. We hold high pressure jobs. We commute in piles of horn honking traffic. Our kids are being compared to the neighbors' kids. We have countless situations that we have no control over. Yet, we hold on to these things and worry endlessly about them and let them affect our lives every single day. All the while, stress management is one of the biggest causes of health problems in our world today. What does that say about us?

If there is one thing aside from your diet and attitude that I can recommend for you to change that will have a HUGE impact on your health, it is managing your stress level. Nothing you are worried about today will matter to you if you find yourself waking up in a hospital bed tomorrow. Get rid of stress!

Chapter 9

How to Party Like a Rock Star...
without being a baby...
or killing yourself

Give a man health and a course to steer, and
he'll never stop to trouble about whether he's
happy or not.
George Bernard Shaw

If you have skipped straight to this chapter, make sure you find me on Facebook or G+ so that we can add you to the invite list for our next bash, you little party animal you.

In all seriousness though, I hope that you weren't thinking that you'd have to give up having fun just because you are getting healthy. Like everything else in your life, there is a way to do it properly. Arming yourself with the know how will keep your stress levels at bay while keeping your party animal status intact.

Alcohol

It's much easier to be a party animal once you have had a few drinks right? WRONG. Alcohol raises the levels of hydrochloric acid in your stomach which directly affects your digestive process. It also makes you think that you can eat an entire chocolate cake and not gain an ounce of weight too. We don't want to knock out all of your fun but if you are a liquor drinker, STOP. Mixed drinks are almost as bad for you as soda is but we aren't going to talk about that yet. Unless you are drinking straight shots, you will most likely be mixing up that liquor with sodas or sugar- laced mixers. STOP STOP STOP. If you must have liquor, make it clear, light in color, and shoot it straight. Come on Rock Star, you asked for this and as my father-in-law always said, "If you are gonna be dumb, you'd better be tough."

Wine

I didn't really fall in love with wine until I began to understand the health benefits that it contained. Because red wines are typically made with the whole grapes including the skins, red wines are packed with antioxidants known as resveratrols. We discussed antioxidants earlier in the book, but just for the sake of repeating the wisdom: Antioxidants can increase the "good" cholesterol in your body and help protect the arteries from damage. Resveratrols also help to eliminate blood clots and they work to inhibit the activities of enzymes in your body that are known to promote cancer growth. Red wine rocks!

White wine, for your information, is made with white grapes and typically, the skins are removed from the light grapes before fermentation. While this sounds like it makes the white wine less healthy, there are still health benefits of drinking white wines. The main benefits of white wines is that they can improve heart health and prevent heart diseases. White wines are also effective in promoting lung health.

Breaking it down, if you really want a drink, make it a tasty wine. Not only will you look smarter to your friends, you will actually be improving your health.

Beer

This may come as a shock to read: beer is actually not bad for you. I would like to add that when I mention beer, I am NOT referring to the watered down crap that the big breweries are putting out there. (You know who they are, so I don't need to name names.) When I discuss beer, I am talking about well made, tasty craft beer.

Not all beer is created equal. Craft beer is quickly gaining popularity in the United States. I personally think this is because people are finally giving a shit about what they are putting into their bodies and they don't want to settle for watered-down crap beer any longer. Watered-down beers are filled with well…WATER for one. They also contain a lot of adjuncts, or fillers. The big beer companies are not in the beer business to enjoy the craft of making beer, they are in it for the money. Most of the large breweries are more concerned about profit margins and ad campaigns than they are concerned with the quality of their ingredients. Craft breweries however, could usually give two shits about profit margins. They have worked hard to perfect their product, and normally are driven by the art of making good beer. Mmmm…beeerrrr.

So, what's in it for you? Craft beer contains 4 base ingredients. Water, malt, hops and yeast. When the brewers are feeling froggy, they will toss in some fruit, spices or herbs to give the beer some added flavors, however you won't typically find chemicals and crap in craft beer. Don't get me wrong, aside from these few pure ingredients, there are also calories and of course once it starts fermentation, you have alcohol, so I am in no way handing you a free pass to drink like a frat boy. I am however debunking some of the crap that has been tossed into the fitness world about beer so that you can be a big girl or big boy and toss back a brew on occasion without feeling bad about it.

Yes, I really meant that beer can be good for you. Craft beer is a significant source of dietary silicon. We NEED silicon in our bodies in order to keep our bones strong. Strong bones keep us from walking like the Hunchback of Notre Dame. Who wants that? Craft beer also contains soluble fiber, vitamins and yes, antioxidants. Mmmmm...beeeerrrr.

Here is the negative that I will give you about beer: it contains yeast. Typically, yeast is a big contributor for making us look like cows. Beer also contains calories. Usually about 150 calories per 12 ounces. Now how many of you head off to your friend's house and only drink ONE beer? Exactly. When you consume more beer, you consume more calories AND more alcohol, which we have already established makes you think that you can eat an entire chocolate cake without gaining a pound, so imagine what it tricks you in to thinking about beer?

Adult drinks of choice as you journey into Health Warriorism: red wine and really good craft beer. End of story.

What if you don't drink alcohol? Please tell me what planet you lived on before you arrived here on earth. I kid, I kid. (not really though)

Fruit juices and prepackaged smoothies

Can you say sugar infested nastiness? Because that is usually what these are. My advice, don't waste your time or your energy on either of these unless you first read the label. You also want to make damn sure that you know what you are looking for/at otherwise, you are going to stay fat and have migraines while you go along pretending that you are healthy.

Soda

Or as you Midwesterners call it, Pop. (I can say that because I used to be Midwest gal.) Repeat after me: "Soda is the devil itself!" I know that some of the nutrition experts say that about sugar so why can't we say it about soda?

There is absolutely NOTHING healthy that comes out of one of those cans or bottles. The crap (IE: caffeine, phosphorus & sodium) can decrease the calcium in your body. Low calcium = Hunchback of Notre Dame syndrome. Let's not even mention the copious amounts of sugar that is found in most sodas. Oh wait, you drink DIET sodas? Yeah, don't go patting yourself on the back that fast. I would like to introduce you to my little friends named Equal, Splenda, Aspartame, Sweet & Low and NutraSweet.

Aspartame was first introduced to the FDA back in 1973 by a gentleman named G.D. Searle. Searle tried eight times to be granted FDA approval on his "miracle sugar."

A scientist named Martha Freeman, who was part of the approval team, declared that there wasn't enough evidence presented by Searle to allow adequate scientific evaluation, and stated that until further testing could be done Aspartame should not be marketed.

Despite Freeman's initial report, Aspartame was approved for use in dry foods in 1974. In 1975, the FDA put together a task force to review the approval of Aspartame based on evidence of the scientific testing being "manipulated." In 1977, the FDA started grand jury proceedings against Searle stating that he knowingly misrepresented the findings and made false statements. There was some back and forth political antics over the next couple of years and in 1980, they finally decided that Aspartame should not be approved for use in foods.

In 1981 a new FDA commissioner was appointed to the FDA. Even though 3 of the 6 scientists decided against approval, the new commissioner overruled the review panel and allowed aspartame into limited foods. In 1983, it was approved for use in beverages and in 1996 aspartame was approved for use without restriction.

Aspartame has a huge list of side effects that the FDA was aware of when it granted approval. Nerve damage, migraine headaches, memory loss, reproductive issues, confusion, brain lesions, blindness, joint pain, bloating, nervous system disorders, hair loss and weight gain.

One of aspartames ingredients converts into formaldehyde.
Formaldehyde is a neurotoxin. And this crap got FDA approval.

NutraSweet and Equal both contain aspartame.
Sweet & Low isn't so sweet either. It contains saccharin which is a compound found in coal tar.

Splenda comes from chlorinating sugar. The end result is sucralose. While the makers of Splenda brag about it being A-OK for diabetics, it is only listed as 98% pure. That other 2%? Heavy metals, methanol and arsenic. Oh yeahhh, let's sprinkle that on everything we eat.

Now that I have scared the crap out of you
I began this chapter by explaining that partying was a necessity to enjoy life. I clearly have told you what to drink and what not to drink. (Wine and Craft Beer = yummy. Soda, Fruit Juice and mixed drinks = bleh) What about the rest of the party? You know, the FOOD?
This is an easy one. Really. You know what you should eat and what you shouldn't. Right? You know how much you should eat as well as how much is too much. So that leaves only one small detail: what in the hell do you do so that you don't turn into a cow when someone invites you to a party?

Here is my list of party survival plans:

✓ When your friend calls to invite you, ask them if you can bring a dish to share. It is a sure fire way to make sure that at least one thing on the buffet is on your "yes" list. If it is going to be a long party, take more than one dish. If your friend declines your offer, take a dish anyway. It is rude to arrive empty handed.

✓ Always eat before you go. Even if the party is a dinner party, have a light snack before you walk out the door. This will ensure that you can keep your head when making food decisions as well as giving you less of a void to fill with high calorie party foods.

✓ Drink plenty of water before, during, and after the party. Water helps to flush toxins out of your system as well as fills your belly. It is good for your skin and your internal organs. Water is a necessity, especially if you are planning to enjoy some good beer or wine.

✓ Pack mints. Mint inhibits hunger. If you are sucking on a peppermint, you are less likely to graze your way through the entire buffet line. Not to mention this will keep your breath minty fresh for any close encounters you may have.

✓ Please for the love of all things festive, do NOT stand at the food area complaining that there is nothing healthy to eat. People don't come to a party to be healthy, they come to have fun. You might stand a better chance for a minty close encounter if you find something better to do with your time than bitch and whine all night.

Being a rock star doesn't have to be stressful. You simply need to arm yourself with knowledge. Now, go grab that little black dress or that kick ass pair of jeans and get out there and party.

Chapter 10

Welcome Warrior

You can not teach a man anything. You can only help him to find it within himself.
Unknown

When I took those first steps on my journey toward better health, I had no clue what I was doing. I spent more time on research than I did on anything else. I read everything that I could get my hands on and followed any author who even remotely resembled someone with food knowledge. I was eager to do things right, and eager to feel healthier. While I still spend many hours on research, I have gained confidence in the decisions that I have made for myself so it has become much easier for me to weed out the bullshit.

Along this road to optimal health, you will encounter haters. (I snagged that word from my kids by the way.) There will be people who think you are crazy. Others who look at you funny and they might even roll their eyes at you. (Happened to me ALL the time.) Your friends will tell you about how wrong you are for doing the things you are doing. My best advice for those moments is to look them in the eye and smile. Thank them for having concern and keep doing exactly what you are doing. You are the only one who knows how you feel and what your body needs.

I am no expert. Sure, my brain is filled with TONS of food knowledge and I know a thing or two about fitness but there are people who are better experts than I am in the field of nutrition and fitness. (They also probably curse less than I do.) Seek them out so that you become confident in your decisions and you aren't just a Wicked Ways Groupie. (although, we LOVE our groupies, we want our followers to be smart and not just mindless sheep.) I have yet to meet a foodie who turns away anyone eagerly seeking better health. We LOVE to hear from you.

I made the decision to go completely plant based. It was a no brainer for me. I realize that it may not be a no brainer for everyone though. As I stated at the very beginning of this book, YOU are in charge of your journey and I encourage you to continue moving forward from here. Making the decisions that are right for you. Sometimes, you may start down a path and realize that it's not exactly the right one for you. Step back, regroup and then move forward in a better direction. We all make mistakes and have to figure things out.

There are countless resources online (remember that some of my favs are listed in the back of this book) that offer more knowledge for you. We frequently host fitness and food challenges on our web site www.OurWickedWays.com, where you can join us for craziness like: The Ten Day Vegan Challenge, Yoga a Day Challenge, Mile A Day Challenge, The Plank Challenge, 5 Minute Meditations, Recipe swaps and our favorite-Google Hang Outs – where you can get face to face with us as well as some of our favorite experts.

The big message: Don't stop here.

You are armed with enough information to drastically change your health. You have enough knowledge at your fingertips to cure yourself from disease, improve chronic conditions and make yourself a true health warrior.

Repeat after me:
I Got This!

Chapter 11
My favorite things

Our greatest happiness does not depend on the condition of life in which chance has placed us, but is always the result of a good conscience, good health, occupation, and freedom in all just pursuits.
Thomas Jefferson

I have been collecting many resources as I traverse the road to better health. I have tried to organize them here so that my favorite things might be able to become your favorite things. Please keep in mind that my journey has been MY journey, not yours. I am not endorsing any of these items personally with statements stating that they are the best of anything, they are simply what I LOVE. As always, remember that YOU are in charge of your health as well as all of the decisions regarding your health.

Nutrition & Diet Knowledge Books:

China Study   by T. Colin Campbell

Whole by T. Colin Campbell

Both of these books by T. Collin Campbell are packed with scientific proofs gathered from years of study by one of nutritions greatest voices. While they are a bit big for an average gobble up reading session, you can not find a better source for nutrition knowledge.

Skinny Bitch   by Rory Freedman & Kim Barnouin

Skinny Bitch was my first real nutrition book. Rory Freedman and Kim Barnouin attack nutrition with such raw truth and emotion that you can't ignore the message. Content warning: the language in the Skinny Bitch books can sometimes be harsh. It is part of the charm. Really.

Cook Books:

The Happy Herbivore Cookbooks   by Lindsay Nixon
Lindsay Nixon is by far one of my favorite plant based chefs. Her recipes are easy to follow, quick to prepare and are beyond tasty. The Happy Herbivore cookbooks are all packed with amazing recipes and beautiful photos. The main thing that I love about Lindsay and her recipes is that she uses regular ingredients that can be found at a common grocery store. Make sure that you check out her website too: www.happyherbivore.com Lindsay has a great meal plan offer available that delivers a weekly meal plan and grocery list right to your email box for next to nothing in cost. (at the time of this writing, it was only $5 per week)

The Sexy Vegan   by Brian Patton
Boys, this is the cook book for you! Slapped full of flavor packed, plant based recipes, Brian really knows how to keep taste buds happy. His book is packed with non-girlie recipes like cocktails named: The Kucklehead and The Bloodbath. He has an entire section devoted to no-meat meat including some to die for "meat"balls as well as a section for snacks that are tough enough for the most edgy football fan.

Movies

Fast Food Nation 2006 Food Matters 2008
Vegucated   2010
Earthlings   2005

Magazines

VegNews
Natural Health

Apps, Sites & Techie Love:

www.OurWickedWays.com - Shelah's health site that is packed FULL of additional resources and information to help you continue on your journey.

www.Happyherbivore.com

www.nomeatathlete.com

www.blytheraw.com

Run Keeper
We use this app to track our routes, mileage and pace for all of our runs. There is great online tracking available and it allows you to view friends activity as well.

 Nike +
Much like Run Keeper mentioned above. We LOVE the challenge feature that Nike+ has.

Zen Labs 5K & 10K apps
I have personally used both of these apps to train for various distances for running. The 5k app is a great place to start your interval training as you work into running.

Yoga Glo

Yoga Glo is a yogis dream for an at home practice. For a small fee each month, you are given access to countless online practices. You can select classes based on time limit, skill level or area of work.

Tools of the Trade:

Vitamix

This is the one appliance that I would highly recommend for anyone who is serious about their health. https://secure.vitamix.com/Classic-Series.aspx?COUPON=%2006-007312

Luna Sandals

We are Luna junkies at our house. These are great sandals which are modeled after the sandals worn by the Tarahumara tribes of South America. Comfortable for walking and running. www.Lunasandals.com

Road ID

 This is a must have piece of gear for any person with a brain. Road ID is the cool kids ID bracelet of our time. Road ID can be customized to include any information that you would like. We highly recommend that you use your name, birth year (not the full date and a couple of emergency contact phone numbers. It will give you and your loved ones a peace of mind when you head out on adventures. http://www.roadid.com/?referrer=8472

Sources

Breaking the Food Seduction: The Hidden Reasons Behind Food
Cravings 2003 Dr. Neal Barnard M.D.

Diet For New America 1987 John Robbins

Whole: Rethinking the Science of Nutrition 2012
T. Colin Campbell

Skinny Bitch 2005
Rory Freedman and Kim Barnouin

The China Study 2006
T. Colin Campbell, Thomas M. Campbell, Howard Lyman & John
Robbins

The American Journal Of Medicine
Volume 126, Issue 5, Pages 411-419, May 2013
http://www.amjmed.com/article/S0002-9343(13)00080-6/abstract

Live Science
http://www.livescience.com/6072-beer-good-bones.html accessed
6-15-2013

Top of the Hops
http://www.topofthehopsbeerfest.com/biloxi/the-top-ten-reasons-
why-you-should-drink-craft-beer accessed 9-4-13

The only person you are destined to become is the person you decide to be.
— Ralph Waldo Emerson

Be fierce. Be happy. Be warriors.
- Shelah Davis

This book has been 2 years in the making for me. Several people crossed my path that have influenced my words, my thoughts and my life while this book was in its rather lengthy stage of creation. I would like to take a moment to send up my gratitude and love for all that they have done and continue to do for me.

To all of my readers, no matter how you happened by this book, you are holding on to a piece of my soul. I thank you for being brave enough to take your first steps, for knowing how to laugh and most of all, for wanting to listen. Without each of you, I would lose my purpose. May you all be true warriors on your journey.

To my friends who have stood by me while I furiously work to change the world. Thank you for believing in me and for proudly waving your pompoms when I have needed it most.

To my sweet editor and friend, Miguel. You and your magic red pen have always been gentle while keeping me inside the grammatical lines. Thank you for never making me deter from who I am during this process.

To my dear friend Kelly, no matter what I have thrown at you, you have always managed to capture the very essence of who I am through your exceptional skills as a graphic designer. You are indeed a fabulous magician as well as a truly wonderful friend. Thank you for always making me look fabulous and fun.

To my sister, who is quite possibly my most insane and best cheerleader. You have never wavered in your faith of me. Despite the many ledges that I walked out onto, I have always known that you would never let me fall but rather you would help me to know that I could indeed fly.

To my Daddy. Thank you for instilling in me, the belief that I could indeed accomplish anything that I set my mind to and for always showing me how to love people without reservation. It is thorough your eyes that I see exactly the path that I am meant to follow. I am certainly following my dreams.

To my angel Momma. Without you, this book would never be what it is. Thank you for being a warrior and for showing me how to fight for what I want and the things that I believe in. You were always filled with grace, beauty and fierceness that can't be matched. I miss you more than I ever thought possible.

To my kids. You three are what keeps me striving to be a better human every single day.

And finally, to my husband. I didn't know it at the time but the day I met you was actually the beginning of my biggest and best adventure. You have taught me how to love and to live with pure joy and unbridled passion. You are my everything.

www.ingramcontent.com/pod-product-compliance
Lightning Source LLC
Chambersburg PA
CBHW020528290526
45786CB00002B/794